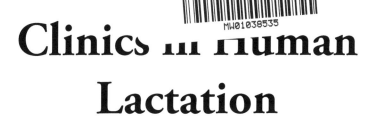

Clinics in Human Lactation

Pumps and Pumping Protocols

Marsha Walker, RN, IBCLC

Breast Pumps and Pumping Protocols
Marsha Walker, RN, IBCLC

Praeclarus Press, LLC

2504 Sweetgum Lane
Amarillo, Texas 79124 USA
806-367-9950
www.PraeclarusPress.com

DISCLAIMER

The information contained in this publication is advisory only and is not intended to replace sound clinical judgment or individualized patient care. The author disclaims all warranties, whether expressed or implied, including any warranty as the quality, accuracy, safety, or suitability of this information for any particular purpose.

ISBN: 9781939807991

Table of Contents

Part 1. Background

Chapter 1. Introduction

Breast pumps have been used for hundreds of years to assist mothers in removing milk from their breasts, providing breastmilk during separations, treating engorgement, or everting flat nipples. Pumping milk is a very personal behavior for most women and often quite subjective. Maternal preferences for manual or powered, double or single pumps reflect the interdependent needs of mother and child, the circumstances that suggest or require pumping, and the affordability of the pump. An employed mother may decide a double electric breast pump is the best option, while a stay-at-home mom may have enough spare moments for a slower single, manual breast pump. Mothers describe their ideal breast pump as one that is inexpensive and works efficiently and comfortably. They want a pump that is easy to assemble, easy to use, and easy to keep clean. Two of the most important features of a breast pump are how much milk can be expressed and how much time it will take to do so.

Walker (1992) conducted an informal survey with more than 200 mothers regarding breast pump usage and opinions. A breast pump was rated highly if it:

- Worked quickly––(less than 20 minutes total)

- Obtained two or more ounces of milk from each breast

- Did not cause pain.

The mothers in this survey utilized several techniques to reduce pumping times and to increase the volume of milk per pumping session. In other words, they added interventions to make the pumps work better. Many mothers expressed the most milk before or after the first morning feeding, when the breasts were reported to be fullest (and intramammary pressure was the highest). The pumped milk volume decreased steadily throughout the day. Many mothers mentioned that if they were not relaxed or if they were uncomfortable or felt rushed, their output dropped by one-third to one-half the usual amount. The majority of mothers used one or more techniques to increase pumping efficiency. The two most frequently mentioned techniques were eliciting the milk-ejection reflex before starting to pump and massaging the breast while pumping. Both techniques reduced the time needed to pump and increased milk output. Some mothers were able to double the amount pumped by using both of these techniques at each pumping session. When looking at breast pump reviews on the Internet, the powered or electric models seemed to receive far more favorable reviews than did the manual models. This was often due to their ease of use and greater efficiency. A few manual breast pumps were given good reviews. The performance features mothers mention in on-line reviews include comfort, ease of milk expression, and pumps that can be easily and quickly cleaned.

The use of breast pumps is becoming more and more common. Data from the Infant Feeding Practices Study II in the United States showed that 85% of breastfeeding mothers in a sample of 1,564 had successfully expressed milk since their infant was born (Labiner-Wolfe, Fein, Shealy, Wang, 2008). Reasons for milk expression that mothers described were to allow someone else to feed the infant and to have an emergency supply on hand for situations such as unplanned separations. Maternal employment was the characteristic that was most strongly associated with expressing milk. Mothers of older infants also expressed to have milk to mix with cereal or other foods. Electric pumps were most frequently used, followed by manual pumps, hand expression, and a combination of electric and battery pump. Less than 2% of mothers used only a battery-powered pump. Similar results were seen in an Australian study of 587 mothers (Perth Infant Feeding Study II - 2002–2004). By six months postpartum, 83.8% of mothers had expressed milk. Mothers who expressed breastmilk in this study were less likely to stop breastfeeding before six months compared with mothers who had never expressed milk (Win, Binns, Zhao, Scott & Oddy, 2006). The authors speculated that the appropriate use of expressed breastmilk could be a means to help mothers achieve six months of exclusive breastfeeding, while giving them more lifestyle options. A survey of breastfeeding women done after the first three weeks of breastfeeding found that mothers who reported expressing milk were 75% less likely to discontinue breastfeeding within the first 12 weeks postpartum than women who did not express breast milk (Schwartz et al., 2002). Binns and colleagues (2006) found that the proportion of mothers who expressed breastmilk had almost doubled between the first Perth Infant Feeding Study conducted in 1992–1993 and the second Perth Infant Feeding Study done a decade later (Binns, Win, Zhao, & Scott, 2006). The majority of mothers in this study expressed breastmilk to manage breastfeeding problems. The authors account for the increase in pump usage through several factors:

• An increase in employed mothers.

• Improved breast pump technology.

- An increased emphasis on exclusive breastfeeding.

- A possible shift in how breastfeeding difficulties are being managed by healthcare providers.

Geraghty and colleagues (2005) looked at the pumping rates of 346 mothers of singleton infants, multiple infants, and preterm infants. Seventy-seven percent of these mothers pumped milk at some point in time during the first six months postpartum. Feeding only at the breast during early postpartum time points was associated with a longer duration of human milk feeding. This most likely emphasizes the importance of getting preterm and multiple infants to the breast as early and as often as possible during the first weeks after birth.

Pumping for some mothers can be an integral part of being able to extend the length of time that an infant is breastfed or receives human milk. In a study of 903 mothers, nearly all had expressed milk (98%), with the most frequent reason being insufficient milk or to make more milk (Clemons & Amir, 2010). Mothers also described pumping to relieve engorgement and to store extra milk. The second most frequent reason for pumping was the return to work. Most women used electric breast pumps and preferred this method to the use of hand pumps or hand expressing. However, only 21% used a double pumping system, despite the fact that pumping both breasts simultaneously is more efficient by more than three hours per week in exclusively pumping mothers (Groh-Wargo et al., 1995; Zinaman, Hughes, Queenan, Labbok, & Albertson, 1992). Although a high use of hand expression was found in this study, very few women preferred this method.

Buckley (2009) looked at the impact of breast pump technology on lactation consultant practice, as well as some of the reasons that breastfeeding mothers desire to use a breast pump. Several themes were derived from this qualitative study.

- Many mothers feel that a breast pump is a necessity if they are to successfully breastfeed their infants. Mothers are inundated with the idea that breast pumps are a normal and accepted part of breastfeeding. Breast pumps appear as a component on layette lists, are present on baby registries, and are received at baby showers. Online blogs and reviews of breast pumps are abundant, as are Internet videos of pumps and how to use them. Mothers wish to have information on breast pumps and ask that this be provided in prenatal classes and in literature distributed during the prenatal period. Many hospitals provide lists of where breast pumps can be purchased or rented, or provide this service themselves. Hospital gift shops may carry pumps, as well as maternity stores, maternity and childcare catalogs, and large toy stores. Breast pumps may be visible in postpartum rooms in the hospital or are readily available if needed. The pervasiveness of pumps could give the impression that if one intends to breastfeed, then a pump is necessary to accomplish one's breastfeeding goals. Some healthcare providers feel that breast pumps have gone from a tool to remedy breastfeeding problems to a piece of technology that reinforces the separation of mother and baby and the demotion of feeding directly at the breast.

• Healthcare providers may be drifting towards over-dependence on breast pumps, causing them to lose the skill of solving breastfeeding problems or being able to teach hand expression. On a bustling and fast paced hospital maternity unit, there may not be the time or personnel needed to properly assess and remedy early breastfeeding challenges. Some hospitals lack the recommended ratio of international board certified lactation consultants (IBCLCs),[1] making pumps an attractive option for busy staff to use in solving issues related to non-latching or non-nursing infants, flat nipples, excessive infant weight loss, etc. Lactation consultants may prematurely turn to pumps in lieu of developing or using assessment and clinical skills in the early management of breastfeeding.

• The increased use of breast pumps seems to parallel the rise in interventions used during childbirth. The cascade of multiple technological interventions experienced during childbirth is thought to contribute to some of the breastfeeding problems seen early in the postpartum period. Clinicians can choose the option of having the mother hand express colostrum and spoon feed it to infants during the first 48 hours, as an alternative to using a pump, as sometimes it is difficult to capture the small amount of colostrum that is in the pump. Colostrum can stick to the sides of the collection container. Breast pumps often become a necessity, however, for either initiating and/or protecting the milk supply during the time it takes to rectify these problems. For example:

  ▷ Large amounts of intravenous fluids (IV) given to the mother during labor can contribute to excess interstitial fluid and an edematous areola, making it difficult for a newborn to latch to the breast (Cotterman, 2004). Placing a pump on an edematous areola

---

1   http://www.ilca.org/files/USLCA/Resources/Publications/IBCLC_Staffing_Recommendations_July_2010.pdf

may actually exacerbate this problem, as nipples swell during pumping (Wilson-Clay & Hoover, 2002). Vacuum from the pump attracts more fluid into the areolar tissue beneath the flange, encouraging this tissue to envelop the nipple, sometimes giving the appearance of a flat or inverted nipple.

▷ Large amounts of IV fluids given to the laboring mother may inflate the birth weight of the infant (Noel-Weiss, Woodend, Peterson, Gibb, & Groll, 2011). When diuresis of this excess fluid occurs, it may be mistaken for excessive weight loss, leading to unnecessary formula supplementation and further difficulty with latching from the use of an artificial nipple. Displacement of sucking from the breast may result in disinterest in feeding and difficulty latching, necessitating pump usage. Iatrogenic problems often lead to the true need for expressing milk.

▷ Receipt of pitocin (synthetic oxytocin), with its anti-diuretic effect favoring water retention, may further contribute to congestion in the areola and latch difficulty. Breast pumps should not be placed on an edematous areola in an effort to evert the nipple or remove colostrum/milk from the breast.

▷ Epidural analgesia and narcotics given to the laboring mother may affect early feeding behaviors (Wiklund, Norman, Uvnäs-Moberg, Ransjö-Arvidson, & Andolf, 2009), resulting in an excessively sleepy infant who does not give clear feeding cues and fails to latch to the breast or latches for only brief periods of time. If this persists, especially after hospital discharge, a breast pump is often used to support milk production. Infants whose mothers had an epidural and develop a fever greater than 101°F have been shown to have a two- to six-fold increased risk of adverse outcomes, such as low Apgar scores, assisted ventilation, early onset seizures, and hypotonia (Greenwell, Wyshak, Ringer, Johnson, Rivkin, & Lieberman, (2012). These are all side effects that could compromise early breastfeeding and result in the need to express milk for an infant having difficulty feeding from the breast.

▷ Vacuum extraction may result in poor early breastfeeding behavior (Hall et al., 2002). Infants unable to latch to the breast or sustain sucking leave the mother vulnerable to insufficient milk, engorgement, and mastitis.

• Breast pumps often represent a way for mothers to control the feeding situation, especially if there are problems. Mothers frequently use or purchase a breast pump due to their concern over not having enough milk, whether or not this is actually the case. Sometimes, a pump is substituted for an assessment by an expert. Mothers may lack access to lactation consultants or may wish to solve problems themselves. Some mothers doubt their ability to fully breastfeed their infant without help from technology. Pumping can be scheduled and milk output can be measured, while direct feeding at the breast is "controlled" by the infant's hunger and need for close contact. The extreme control of feedings resides in the situation where mothers choose not to directly breastfeed, but instead to pump milk for all feedings. This is a growing trend with no clear research on why the increase in the phenomena is happening. Mothers have voiced a number of reasons for their choice that included: feared direct breastfeeding, allowed mothers to know exactly how much the baby is getting, promoted more sleep at night since they felt they didn't have to get up as frequently, experienced pain and other problems which precluded feeding directly at breast, may have been victims of sexual abuse, had a baby that never latched, or had an infant with oral, neurological, or other anomalies that prevented direct breastfeeding. These mothers most likely persisted with exclusive pumping, as they appreciated the value of human milk for their infant and wanted the child to have breastmilk for its nutritional and immunological properties. Exclusive pumping is more work for the mother, but it leaves the option open of direct breastfeeding later on for some mothers, depending on the situation.

• Breast pumps are an important and appropriate tool in a number of situations, such as premature infants and employed mothers. Such situations create a dependency on a pump to assure that breastmilk is available for many months, irrespective of the infant being present at the breast. It requires a commitment and dedication on the part of the mother to invest her time in assuring that her infant receives as much of her milk as possible.

Exclusive pumping is less expensive than feeding infant formula to a baby. A mother who is exclusively pumping could expect to pay between $450 and $720 to rent a hospital grade, double pumping, electric breast pump for a year. The collection kit would cost approximately $56, and 10 bottles would cost about $50—totaling $556–$826. Costs for just the infant formula to feed a baby for one year would total between $1250 and $2600, depending on the type of formula used. This does not include bottles, nipples, or the increased health expenses experienced by infants who are exclusively formula-fed.

Breast pumps have a role in enabling mothers to prolong the amount of time an infant receives human milk, with some mothers crediting the use of a breast pump with their ability to avoid premature weaning. Breast pumps have a drawback in that they represent a way to "promote breastfeeding," while avoiding more difficult, divisive, and stubborn social and economic issues. From a policy-making or employer standpoint, breast pumps may seem a less expensive and easier way to mollify employees without addressing the underlying issue of paid maternity leave and other social ills that separate mothers and infants or create disparities in care for low-income women.

Chapter 2. History of Breast Pumps

Medical literature cites breast pump use as early as the mid 1500s (Fildes, 1986), although instruments for solving breastfeeding problems have probably been around for much longer than this. Sucking glasses (Figure 2.1) were used to relieve engorgement, express milk during mastitis and cracked nipples, and evert flat nipples. Mothers could use these instruments by themselves, rather than having to rely on a birth attendant or other person to assist in milk removal. If a mother did not possess a sucking glass, she could fill a glass or glass vial with scalding hot water (L in Figure 2.1), empty the water out, and place the mouth of the vial over her nipple, areola, and breast, which would draw out the nipple and encourage milk flow. Mothers did not express large quantities of milk to store for future use, but used these early pumps to remedy acute breastfeeding problems. Vacuum in early breast pumps was generated by the midwife or the mother sucking on the end of a tube (Figure 2.1 and Figure 2.2).

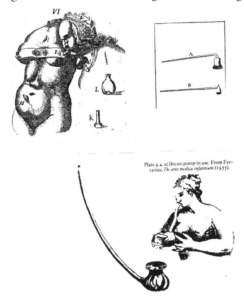

Plate 4.4. a) Breast pump in use. From Ferrarius, *De arte medica infantium* (1577).

Figure 2.1. Sucking Pipes and Glasses From the 1500s and 1600s.

Source: Ferrarius O. De arte medica infantium, de Marchettis 1577; Scultetus J. The chyrurgeon's storehouse, J. Starkey, 1674

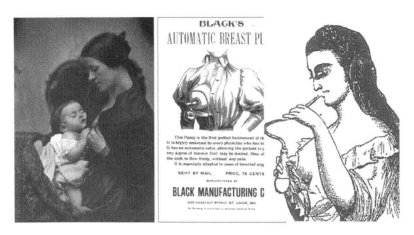

Figure 2.2. Blown Glass Collection Containers Appeared in the 1700s and 1800s.

Vacuum in the "next generation" of breast pumps was accomplished by pulling on a plunger, although there was no easy way to regulate the amount of vacuum these pumps were able to generate. Metal parts became available and were more durable, leaving many operating examples of the types of pumps that started to be used during the 1700s and 1800s (Figure 2.3). It was still difficult for a mother to express milk by herself.

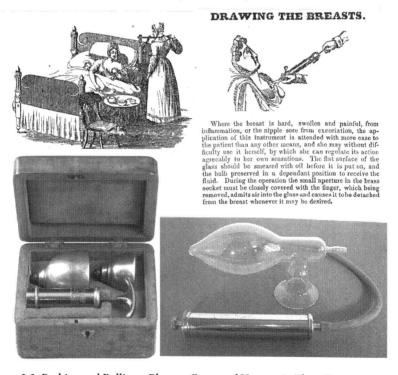

Figure 2.3. Pushing and Pulling a Plunger Generated Vacuum in These Pumps.

The "bicycle horn" breast pump (Figure 2.4) became very popular worldwide in the mid 1800s and can still be found in use today. In these pumps, vacuum is generated by squeezing and releasing a rubber bulb, while milk collects in a collection reservoir. Sometimes the amount collected is as little as one-half ounce.

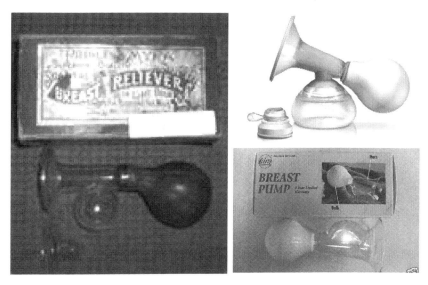

Figure 2.4. Bicycle Horn Breast Pump Generates Vacuum by Squeezing and Releasing a Rubber Bulb

Some manufacturers separated the rubber bulb from the collection container by attaching the bulb to a length of tubing, with a feeding bottle as a collecting container (Figure 2.5). This modification prevented the milk from backing up into the rubber bulb and becoming contaminated. Vacuum was still poorly controlled with these types of pumps, even with the addition on one brand of pump of a vacuum knob on the rubber bulb similar to that on a blood pressure cuff.

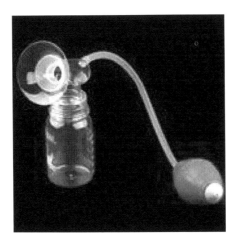

Figure 2.5. A Modified Rubber Bulb Pump

On June 20, 1854, the *United States Patent Office* issued Patent No. 11,135 to O.H. Needham[2] for a breast pump (Figure 2.6). The vacuum on this pump was generated by pushing on a bellows. The flange was made of rubber and was claimed to be flexible enough to collapse on the breast. This was different from the rigid glass flange other pumps of the era provided. *Scientific American* (1863) credits L.O. Colbin as the inventor and patent applicant of a breast pump adapted from a cow milker (Figure 2.7). In 1924, chess master *Edward Lasker,* who was trained as an engineer, patented an electric breast pump that had adjustable suction and cycling (Figure 2.8). This pump claimed to operate at 40–80 cycles per minute and provide vacuum that could be adjusted from a low of 25 to 50 mmHg to a high of 126 to 229 mmHg.[3]

2 http://www.google.com/patents?id=fSVNAAAAEBAJ&printsec=abstract&zoom=4#v=onepag e&q&f=false

3 http://www.freepatentsonline.com/1644257.pdf

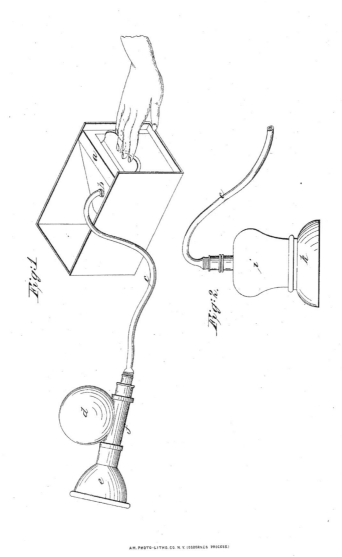

Figure 2.6. Hand Operated Bellows Pump, 1854

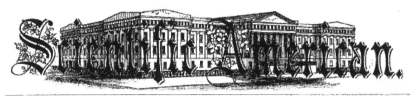

WEEKLY JOURNAL OF PRACTICAL INFORMATION IN ART, SCIENCE, MECHANICS, CHEMISTRY AND MANUFACTURES.

VOL. VIII.—NO. 4 }
(NEW SERIES.)

NEW YORK, JANUARY 24, 1863.

{SINGLE COPIES SIX CENTS.
$3 PER ANNUM—IN ADVANCE.

Fruits of Yankee Energy

When it was first proposed to accomplish the milking of cows by machinery, the thing was looked upon as an utter impossibility. So far from the public entertaining the proposition seriously, they only laughed at it as being the very acme of absurdity—invention in fact run mad. However, the shrewd projectors of this scheme believed in the old saw, "let them laugh who win," and consequently set about accomplishing their object without the least delay. This invention—published in the Scientific American, Vol. III (new series), page 4—has been greatly improved since that time, and we think it is now the best, as it is the only machine of its class in use.

The operation of it will be readily understood by referring to our illustration. The four elastic thimbles encircling the teats of the cow's udder connect by apertures at their bases, with the concave metal pan. Attached to this metal pan there is an india-rubber diaphragm or sheet which by operating the levers grasped by the milker gives a remittent action, and produce a partial vacuum in the metal pan in obedience to natural laws; the milk then flows in a stream into the pail beneath, through a valve just over the end of the elastic pipe leading to the same. When the milking is concluded, the operator merely lets go of the handles, and the machine then remains suspended under one arm by the straps over the breast and shoulder, and the milkman is free to go anywhere unembarrassed by the instrument. The whole affair is very light and simple in action, and can be readily taken apart and cleaned. For a view of the internal construction of this invention see the "breast-pump," illustrated on this page; they are alike.

A portion of this invention was patented in this country, through the Scientific American Patent Agency, and also in England, some time ago; but it has recently been improved and other patents are now pending before the U. S. Patent Office. A stock company has been formed in England, with a capital of $130,000, to work this patent; and the British cows will have the satisfaction of being deprived of their lacteal product by a Yankee machine in the shortest possible space of time. Persons who desire farther information in regard to the

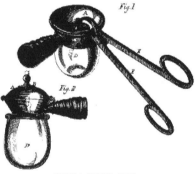

THE CELEBRATED PATENT COW-MILKER.

terms of territorial rights should address Kershaw & Colvin, patentees and manufacturers, 118 North Broad street, Philadelphia, Pa.

COLVIN'S BREAST PUMP.

This engraving, which we have previously referred to, represents a breast pump, such as is used for obvious purposes by nurses and the medical faculty. It is upon the same principle as the "cow-

milker" illustrated in the preceding engraving. In figure 1, A is the elastic india-rubber diaphragm attached to the metal disk, B, and to the metallic flange C. To the latter is secured the glass chamber, D. A corrugated elastic rubber-pipe, a, is coupled to the nozzle, b, and is attached at the other extremity to the breast. Fig. 2 shows the pump in section with the diaphragm in dotted lines at the bottom, and also stretched to its fullest extension on top. The small sheet-rubber valve, c, is also shown, which closes the connection between the glass chamber and the breast. It will be seen that by working the two handles, F F, in Fig. 1, that a remitting action of the diaphragm is produced which is similar to nature's operations, and which is attended with the result it is desired to attain. This pump is the invention of L. O. Colvin, of Philadelphia. Application for a patent is now pending through the Scientific American Patent Agency. For further information, address Kershaw & Colvin, 118 North Broad street, Philadelphia, Pa.

Foreign Stamp Canceling.—Since the publication of our article on this subject we have been visited with a perfect shower of devices designed to accomplish this result, many of which have shown considerable ingenuity ; thus adding another proof that our inventors are equal to any emergency. There seems to be an objection to implements designed to cut or perforate the stamp, owing chiefly to the fact that they would soon get out of order by the constant and rapid use to which they would be exposed. The simplest plan yet suggested, it seems to us, is that of gumming but half the stamp, allowing the other half to be torn off with facility. In a recent article published on page 42 of our present volume, we suggested the practical difficulties that would attend the introduction of the proposed new stamp, though we regard the remedy as quite simple and liable to few objections. We repeat that what we said on a former occasion, that time and money would be wasted on any plan unless the Government first adopted it. Whoever is lucky enough to convince Uncle Sam of the value of his device, ought to secure it by Letters Patent.

Figure 2.7. Colvin's Breast Pump Adapted From His Cow Milker, 1863

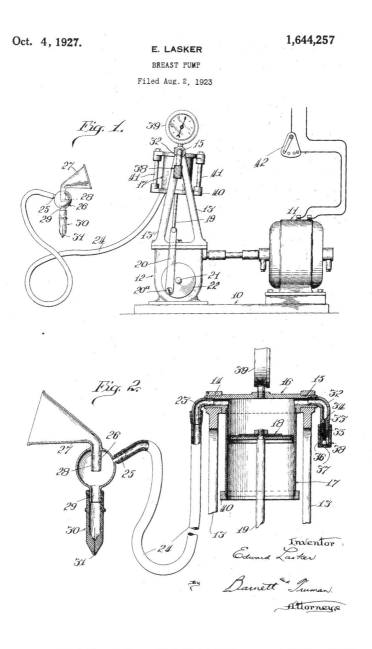

Oct. 4, 1927.

E. LASKER

BREAST PUMP

Filed Aug. 2, 1923

1,644,257

Figure 2.8. Lasker's Electric Pump With Variable Vacuum and Cycling, 1927

In 1956 Einar Egnell published his groundbreaking work, "Viewpoints on what happens mechanically in the female breast during various methods of milk collection." This article provided insight into the technical aspects of milk extraction from the breast and has formed the foundation for breast pump designs. Egnell discussed the concept that a pump does not pump, suck, or pull milk out of the breast. The negative pressure that is generated by a pump reduces resistance to milk outflow from the alveoli, permitting the internal pressure within the breast to push out the milk. The milk-ejection reflex produces an initial rise in the intramammary pressure. Because of the pulsatile nature of oxytocin release and its short half-life, periodic rises in ductal pressure (multiple let downs) reinforce the pressure gradient during the time the breast is being expressed. Milk thus moves from an area of high pressure (within the breast created by the milk ejection reflex) to an area of low pressure (vacuum created by a pump or an infant's mouth).

Egnell based his research on the anatomy and milking of dairy cattle, plus his own experiments with a pump that created periodic and limited phases of negative pressure. Egnell assumed that the milk-secreting alveoli of the breast and the cow udder were similar, even though the two organs are anatomically different and do not drain in the same way. He theorized that the quantity of milk secreted by a breast is regulated by the counterpressure it exerts. This counterpressure rises as milk fills the available space. Egnell thought that milk synthesis ceased when the pressure within the breast reached 28 mmHg, like turning off a faucet. Egnell's pump created a maximum negative pressure of 200 mmHg below atmospheric pressure (760 mmHg). He based this setting on previous research done with an Abt pump (on human mothers), which produced 30 periods of negative pressure per minute and was reported to rupture the nipple skin in every third breast. This type of research would not be permitted today. Placing his settings well below this level to avoid damaging the human nipple, Egnell calculated the difference between the pressure-filled alveoli and his pump's negative pressure as $760 + 28 - 560 = 228$ mmHg. He maintained that when the milk tension within the breast reached 28 mmHg, it reached equilibrium, with the resistance to outflow in the nipple. The milk remained in the breast until negative pressure was experienced by the breast and the positive pressure within overcame the lower pressure generated by the infant's mouth or a breast pump. The difference in pressure caused the milk to flow from an area of high pressure (within the breast) to an area of lower pressure (in the pump). The role of negative pressure or vacuum that is generated by a breast pump serves to reduce the resistance to the outflow of milk from the breast.

Egnell's original pump operated in four phases per cycle, with one cycle lasting from one initiation of suction to the next initiation of suction: (1) a period of increasing suction that is relatively short, (2) a decreasing phase of suction, (3) a resting phase, and (4) a slight amount of positive pressure when the decreased suction phase is finished. This type of suction curve can be seen in present day electric pumps, with various pumps having slightly differing suction curves. Egnell believed that pumping milk mechanically was safer and a better option than expressing milk by hand because he speculated that the "high" positive pressure generated by "squeezing" the breast could damage the internal workings of the breast, such as the alveoli and ducts. He also thought that manual expression would leave too much milk in the breast, a common concern in the dairy industry, where too much residual milk left in the udder after milking added a risk factor for mastitis. However, no research could be located that correlated internal breast damage to hand expression.

Many pump manufacturers still use Egnell's pressure settings as a guide. However, various pumps are capable of generating more suction than stated in his calculations and have the potential to cause damage to the nipple and areolar skin and underlying tissues. Based on Egnell's work, the SMB breast pump (Figure 2.9) became the early standard for electric breast pump design.

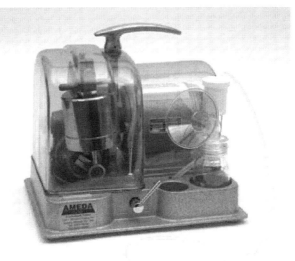

Figure 2.9. The SMB Electric Breast Pump

Breast pumps began to proliferate in the 1980s and 1990s, with manual, battery, and electric pumps offered from many manufacturers. Cylinder pumps consisted of an inner cylinder with a flange that was placed against the breast and an outer cylinder that moved back and forth to generate vacuum (Figure 2.10).

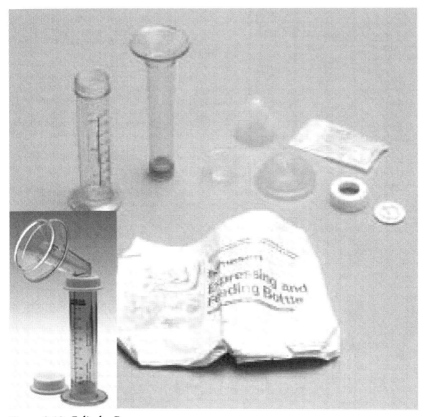

Figure 2.10. Cylinder Pumps

Other hand pumps used a plunger to generate vacuum or handles that were squeezed (Figure 2.11).

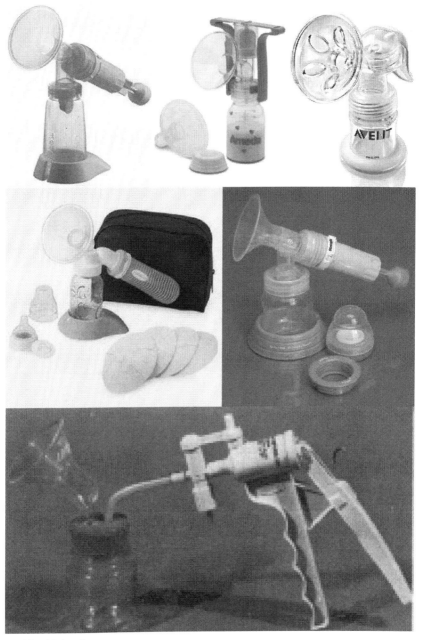

Llyod B hand pump

Figure 2.11. Hand Pumps Using Plungers or Handles

Battery operated pumps came on the market as an option that did not require as much work to use them and as a less expensive option than the larger electric pumps. Many offered AC adapters to save on battery use (Figure 2.12).

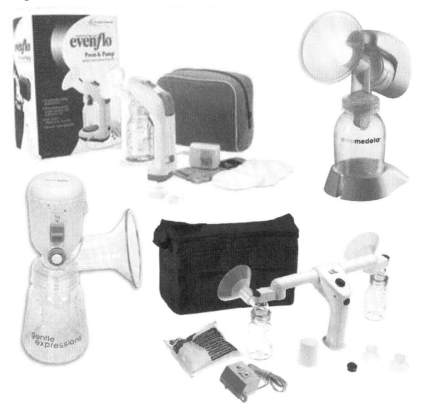

Figure 2.12. Various Battery Operated Pumps

Some of the early, large electric pumps were modifications of equipment used for other medical indications, such as chest aspirators. These generated constant vacuum (not cycled vacuum). Vacuum was initiated when the mother placed her finger over a valve and was released when she lifted her finger (Figure 2.13).

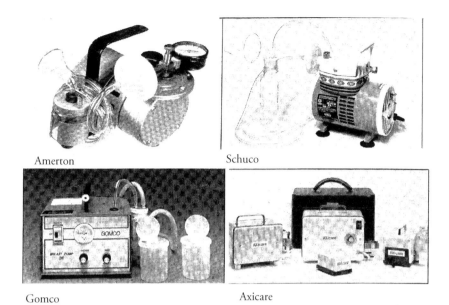

Amerton   Schuco

Gomco   Axicare

Figure 2.13. Modified Aspirators

Small electric pumps were brought to market, with some having double pumping capability. These small pumps sometimes alternated pumping from one breast to the other rather than having the capability of pumping both breasts simultaneously (Figure 2.14).

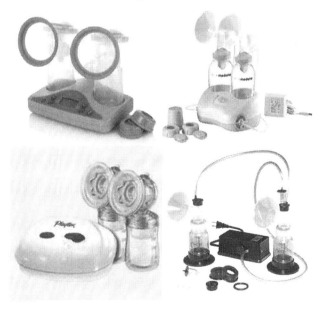

Figure 2.14. Small Electric Pumps

Large electric pumps (sometimes called hospital grade) became available that could be rented (as many were quite expensive to purchase) and were used for mothers of preterm infants, employed mothers, or with conditions that required long term pumping or initiating and maintaining a milk supply in the absence of an infant at breast. These were often multi-user pumps that could be used by more than one mother (Figure 2.15).

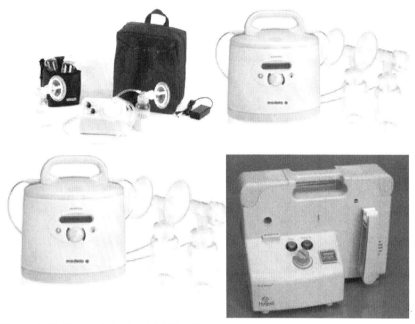

Figure 2.15. Hospital-Grade Multi-User Pumps

Personal-use pumps were marketed as a more efficient alternative to the small electric pumps and a less expensive option than the large hospital-grade or multi-user pumps. These are popular for employed mothers who pump on a daily basis (Figure 2.16).

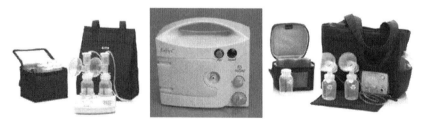

Figure 2.16. Personal-Use Pumps

A number of other miscellaneous pumps have appeared over the years that have other sources of vacuum generation (Figure 2.17).

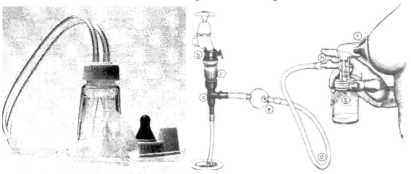

The Ora'lac pump. Vacuum was generated by the mother when she sucked on a length of tubing that was connected to the top of the collecting bottle.

This pump generated vacuum from a stream of water. Vacuum was initiated when the mother placed her finger over a valve and released when she lifted her finger.

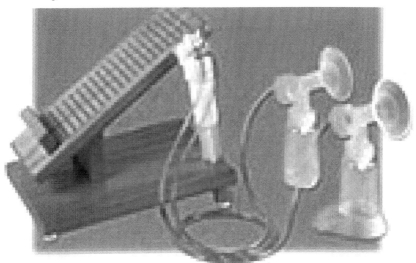

Pedal pump generates vacuum when the mother pushes down and up on a foot pedal.

Figure 2.17. Pumps With Other Vacuum Sources

Dozens of pumps have come and gone over the years, with manufacturers constantly changing features, discontinuing some models, and introducing new ones. No breast pump is as effective as an efficiently nursing infant. The variety of pumps currently on the market can be bewildering to a new mother and confusing to a clinician, especially if knowledge of pumps and pumping is based solely on manufacturers' claims. Pump effectiveness can be highly individual. Clinical experience has shown that some mothers can pump abundant amounts of milk with pumps that are considered to be ineffective and poorly designed, while other mothers have difficulty maintaining good production with the best hospital-grade, multi-user breast pump. Pumping protocols (how the pumps are used) also influence how effective breast pumps will be for mothers.

Chapter 3.
Regulation of Breast Pumps

Breast pumps in the United States are regulated by the Food and Drug Administration's (FDA) Center for Devices and Radiological Health (CDRH).[4] Historically, medical device regulation was very limited under the Food, Drug, and Cosmetic Act of 1938. Amendments were made to this Act in 1976 that established a more rigorous set of regulatory requirements. Devices on the market prior to 1976 did not require FDA review of their safety and effectiveness. The amendments established pathways for bringing new devices onto the market, devised classifications for devices based on risk, and created advisory panels to review the results of pre-market studies (Newburger, 2006). There are three classifications for medical devices, each with its own set of regulatory guidelines:

• Class I. This is the lowest level for devices, with general guidelines that include adherence to good manufacturing practices, labeling regulations, and record keeping by the manufacturer that are designed to provide a basic level of assurance of a safe and effective product. Non-powered breast pumps are classified at this level (Box 3.1).

---

4   http://www.fda.gov/MedicalDevices/ProductsandMedicalProcedures/ HomeHealthandConsumer/ConsumerProducts/BreastPumps/ucm061584.htm

Box 3.1. FDA Classification for Non-Powered Breast Pumps

[Code of Federal Regulations]

[Title 21, Volume 8]

[Revised as of April 1, 2011]

[CITE: 21CFR884.5150]

TITLE 21--FOOD AND DRUGS

CHAPTER I--FOOD AND DRUG ADMINISTRATION
DEPARTMENT OF HEALTH AND HUMAN SERVICES

SUBCHAPTER H--MEDICAL DEVICES

PART 884 -- OBSTETRICAL AND GYNECOLOGICAL DEVICES

Subpart F--Obstetrical and Gynecological Therapeutic Devices

Sec. 884.5150 Nonpowered breast pump.

(a) *Identification.* A nonpowered breast pump is a manual suction device
used to express milk from the breast.

(b) *Classification.* Class I. The device is exempt from the premarket
notification procedures in subpart E of part 807 of this chapter, subject to
the limitations in 884.9, if the device is using either a bulb or telescoping
mechanism which does not develop more than 250 mmHg suction, and the
device materials that contact breast or breast milk do not produce
cytotoxicity, irritation, or sensitization effects.

[45 FR 12684–12720, Feb. 26, 1980, as amended at 61 FR 1124, Jan. 16,
1996; 66 FR 38809, July 25, 2001]

Source: http://www.accessdata.fda.gov/scripts/cdrh/cfdocs/cfcfr/CFRSearch.
cfm?fr=884.5150

- Class II. These devices require more than just general controls.
  Manufacturers may need to provide guidance documents, performance

standards, or some sort of post market surveillance. Powered breast pumps are classified as Class II medical devices.

- Class III. These devices are defined as supporting or sustaining life and require much more extensive study before being allowed on the market.

Before a medical device can be placed on the market, the manufacturer is required to file with the FDA either a Pre-Market Approval or a 510(k) submission. Pre-Market Approvals are filed for complex medical devices, new technology, or new indications for a previously marketed product that raises questions regarding safety and effectiveness. This is an extensive submission, which even requires that the FDA inspect the manufacturing facility and audit some of the clinical testing sites. Breast pumps are approved through the 510(k) application, where the safety and effectiveness of the device is compared to those of a "substantially equivalent" commercial device that is already on the market. The 510(k) process is quick, less costly, and requires little in the way of premarket testing. It does not require that any clinical data be submitted at all. Under the 510(k) requirements, a manufacturer can simply claim that the function of the product, as well as its safety and effectiveness, are equivalent to another similar product that is already on the market. Thus the new product can even be claimed to be substantially equivalent to a product on the market prior to 1976, when less stringent regulations were in effect. Clinicians should be aware that many breast pumps may never have been tested with clinical trials involving mothers to assess the safety and effectiveness of the product. There may be no clinical testing data available from the manufacturer and nothing more than literature making claims regarding the pump for marketing purposes. Box 3.2 is a sample of a 510(k) application for a breast pump and the FDA's response, allowing the pump to be placed on the market. The manufacturer claims that the pump is similar to other pumps already on the market, but the pump seems to have never been tested on mothers in the settings in which it will be used.

Box 3.2. Sample of a 510(K) Submission and the FDA Reply

Design and materials:
All components that may come in contact with the milk are manufactured from materials that meet FDA food contact criteria. The materials that contact the breast have been tested for biocompatibility.

Intended Use:
An electrically powered breast pump with settings, for expressing milk from the breasts of a lactating woman.

Technological Characteristics of the Device:
The Gerber Double Electric Breast Pump is substantially equivalent to other powered breast pumps that are available for commercial distribution. A chart showing the similarities and differences of the proposed powered breast pump and the predicate powered breast pumps follows:

Comparison of Predicate Devices				
	New device	K031614	K022594	K973501
	Gerber DoubleElectric Breast Pump	Medela Pump-in-Style	Playtex Breast Pump	Ameda Egnell Purely Yours
Intended Use:	Express milk	Express milk	Express milk	Express milk
Power Source:	DC	DC	DC	DC
Pump Style:	Diaphragm	Diaphragm	Reciprocating Piston	Reciprocating Piston
Single/double Pumping:	Both	Both	Both	Both
Adjustable Suction Levels:	Yes	Yes	Yes	Yes
Cycle Speed:	Fixed	Variable	Variable	Variable
Overflow Protection:	No	No	Yes	Yes
Highest Vacuum Setting – (mmHg):	240	250	229	170
Lowest Vacuum Setting	0	0	64	31
Active Breast Massage:	Yes	No	Yes	No
Software (microchip)	Yes	Yes	Yes	Yes

Discussion of Non-clinical Tests:
Bench testing of the device has demonstrated that the Gerber Double Electric Breast pump meets established requirements when used in the manner and environment specified in product labeling.

Discussion of clinical tests performed:
No clinical tests have been conducted on this device.

Conclusion:
The Gerber Double Electric Breast Pump is safe and effective for its intended use of milk expression and is substantially equivalent to the predicate devices.

 DEPARTMENT OF HEALTH & HUMAN SERVICES   Public Health Service

Food and Drug Administration
9200 Corporate Boulevard
Rockville MD 20850

DEC 15 2004

Gerber Products Company
% Ms. Chantel Carson
Manager
Underwriters Laboratories, Inc.
Northbrook Division
333 Pfingsten Road
NORTHBROOK IL 60062-2096

Re: K043098
Trade/Device Name: Gerber Double
        Electric Breast Pump
Regulation Number: 21 CFR 884.5160
Regulation Name: Powered breast pump
Regulatory Class: II
Product Code: 85 HGX
Dated: November 24, 2004
Received: November 30, 2004

Dear Ms. Carson:

We have reviewed your Section 510(k) premarket notification of intent to market the device referenced above and have determined the device is substantially equivalent (for the indications for use stated in the enclosure) to legally marketed predicate devices marketed in interstate commerce prior to May 28, 1976, the enactment date of the Medical Device Amendments, or to devices that have been reclassified in accordance with the provisions of the Federal Food, Drug, and Cosmetic Act (Act) that do not require approval of a premarket approval application (PMA). You may, therefore, market the device, subject to the general controls provisions of the Act. The general controls provisions of the Act include requirements for annual registration, listing of devices, good manufacturing practice, labeling, and prohibitions against misbranding and adulteration.

If your device is classified (see above) into either class II (Special Controls) or class III (Premarket Approval), it may be subject to such additional controls. Existing major regulations affecting your device can be found in the Code of Federal Regulations, Title 21, Parts 800 to 898. In addition, FDA may publish further announcements concerning your device in the Federal Register.

Please be advised that FDA's issuance of a substantial equivalence determination does not mean that FDA has made a determination that your device complies with other requirements of the Act or any Federal statutes and regulations administered by other Federal agencies. You must comply with all the Act's requirements, including, but not limited to: registration and listing (21 CFR Part 807); labeling (21 CFR Part 801); good manufacturing practice requirements as set forth in the quality systems (QS) regulation (21 CFR Part 820) and if applicable, the electronic product radiation control provisions (Sections 531-542 of the Act); 21 CFR 1000-1050.

Source: http://www.accessdata.fda.gov/cdrh_docs/pdf4/K043098.pdf

While there are some similarities between pumps that are claimed to be substantially equivalent, there are also some important differences. Also, the manufacturer has chosen the attributes for comparison, which can bias the conclusion of equivalency. Seventy-eight breast pumps have been cleared by the FDA since 1980.[5] Clinicians can check which pumps have been cleared by the FDA and view the manufacturer's 510(k) application online.[5] Not all breast pumps may be listed, as some of the non-powered breast pumps require only a notification be sent to the FDA that the product will be sold. The FDA maintains a website on breast pumps that provides basic information and resources for both mothers and clinicians.[6]

There may be somewhat of a disconnect when comparing a 510(k) application with the marketing claims that a manufacturer makes about its pump. On the one hand, the pump is said to be substantially equivalent to a competitor's pump in the 510(k) application, but the manufacturer frequently claims in its marketing literature how unique and effective their product is compared to other brands of pumps. There are obviously limitations in the evaluation of breast pumps. Just because a breast pump has received FDA clearance, it does not mean that the pump is effective or will perform as indicated in marketing claims.

The FDA monitors the performance of medical devices through a passive surveillance system, called MedWatch, which allows reports to be filed regarding adverse events and problems with products.[7] Both clinicians and mothers can file adverse event reports to MedWatch and are encouraged to do so. These reports, including the descriptive text of the problem, are entered into the Manufacturer and User Facility Device Experience (MAUDE) database.[8] This database can be searched to see the nature and number of problems experienced with breast pumps. Most likely only a small percentage of such problems are ever reported, but the database gives clinicians an idea of the types of problems mothers encounter with various breast pumps. Brown and colleagues (2005) accessed FDA databases for adverse events reported for breast pumps between 1992 and 2002. There were 37 reports filed between 1992 and 2003. The majority of reports (81%) were for electric or battery-operated pumps. Most of the reports were for malfunctions of the pumps. The most frequently reported problems for electric or battery-operated pumps were pain, soreness, discomfort, and tissue damage. The most common problems reported for manual pumps were tissue damage and infection. Malfunctions were reported related to vacuum that was either inadequate or that could not be released. Pain and tissue damage caused by excessive vacuum or vacuum that was applied for

5   http://www.accessdata.fda.gov/scripts/cdrh/devicesatfda/index.cfm?st=breast%20pumps
6   http://www.fda.gov/MedicalDevices/ProductsandMedicalProcedures/
      HomeHealthandConsumer/ConsumerProducts/BreastPumps/default.htm
7   http://www.fda.gov/Safety/MedWatch/HowToReport/default.htm
8   http://www.accessdata.fda.gov/scripts/cdrh/cfdocs/cfMAUDE/TextSearch.cfm

long periods of time without interruption were reported. Vacuum is needed to create and maintain a pressure gradient to allow milk to flow. However, vacuum that is too high and creates pain can interfere with the let-down reflex and reduce milk output. Vacuum that is too low may result in a pump that creates an inefficient pressure gradient and fails to remove sufficient amounts of milk, jeopardizing the mother's milk supply.

In a search of the MAUDE database from 2005 through 2011, there are a few reports each year of pumps that malfunction or cause injury. However, in 2010 and 2011, there was a tremendous jump in reports for adverse effects in pumps from one manufacturer. Many of these reports were for defective power cords and power supplies that were sparking or catching fire (Box 3.3).

Box 3.3. Adverse Events for Breast Pumps From MAUDE Database 2005 Through 2011

2005	3 complaints were filed for Evenflo (no milk expressed), 1 for Bailey Nurture III (nipple crack), 2 for First Years (pain, malfunction), 2 for Medela (mold in tubing), 2 for Playtex Embrace (nipple wound), 1 for Ameda (outer seal on box was broken)
2006	1 complaint for First Years electric (mold in pump), 1 for Evenflo (cracked nipple, no milk expressed), 1 for Avent Isis IQ Duo (pain and cracked nipple), 1 for Medela Pump in Style (tubing melted in microwave steam bag)
2007	1 complaint was filed for Playtex (injury, nipple crack), 1 for Medela (mother's nipple got stuck in flange), 1 for Evenflo (pain, poor milk expression), 1 for Avent manual (areolar lacerations from "petals" on flange)
2008	1 complaint for Egnell (injury)
2010	81 complaints were filed for Medela (electrical malfunctions, melted electrical parts, sparking)
2011	112 complaints for Medela (mostly power supply sparking, fires, some complaints about injury to nipples, and mold in the pump), 1 complaint for Simplisse (difficulty expressing with manual pump)

Source: http://www.accessdata.fda.gov/scripts/cdrh/cfdocs/cfMAUDE/TextSearch.cfm

The FDA has issued warning letters to various pump manufacturers over the years for various infractions. The FDA issued a warning letter to Medela in 2011.[9]Medela issued a voluntary recall on some of its Pump in Style Advanced pumps in 2010. [10]

If mothers contact the customer service department of a pump manufacturer with a complaint, the complaint is supposed to be logged, rectified, and reported to the FDA. The FDA issued a warning letter to Evenflo in 2009 regarding "failure to review and evaluate all complaints" and for failing "to establish medical device reporting procedures for your breast pumps." The FDA reviewed 37 complaints. Of those, 18 were not investigated by the company, including at least three reports of women receiving an electrical shock when using the breast pumps.[11] A warning letter was issued in 2003 to The First Years for marketing a breast pump without pre-market notification, as the FDA requires breasts pumps to be cleared prior to being placed on the market.[12]

There are most likely a much larger number of problems with breast pumps that are never reported to the FDA, either because clinicians and mothers are not aware of the complaint process or due to the idea that problems with pumps are a normal part of using the devices. This under-reporting is evident in looking at reviews of breast pumps on Internet websites. Mothers list numerous problems with many brands of pumps, sometimes receiving two or more replacement part or pumps from the manufacturer. There are many more reports of pump problems on these Internet sites than are ever reported to the FDA.

Sometimes, however, it is difficult to sort out if the pump is faulty or if it is how the pump is used that contributes to the complaint by the mother. Mothers may have unrealistic expectations of what some pumps can do or may be using the pump in a manner that can damage nipple tissue. On the other hand, obvious mechanical shortcomings leave no doubt where the problem lies. The reports sent to the FDA are not verified by the FDA, nor do they establish cause and effect. It is important to report these problems to the FDA and to the manufacturer, since the manufacturer is required by the FDA to use this information to improve their product and remediate the reported problems, as well as report the problems to the FDA. Mothers and clinicians should report pump problems both to the manufacturer and to the FDA's MedWatch system. To report pump problems to the FDA's

9   http://www.fda.gov/ICECI/EnforcementActions/WarningLetters/ucm245251.htm
10 http://www.medelabreastfeedingus.com/product-returns
11 http://www.fda.gov/ICECI/EnforcementActions/WarningLetters/2009/ucm181777.htm
12 http://www.fda.gov/ICECI/EnforcementActions/EnforcementStory/
    EnforcementStoryArchive/ucm095264.htm

MedWatch system, mothers and clinicians can submit them online at http://www.fda.gov/Safety/MedWatch/default.htm, fax them to the FDA at 1–800–322–0178, or call them in at 1–800–FDA–1088.

Safety Issues

There are a number of safety issues related to breast pumps that include assuring that the pump does not generate an unsafe level of vacuum, the vacuum is sufficient to maintain milk production, the pump can be sufficiently cleaned to assure the pumped milk is not contaminated, and the pump does not cause tissue injury or damage. In some reports to the FDA of pump problems, there is a mention of associated mastitis. Foxman and colleagues (2002) followed 946 women for the first three months postpartum. Among the mothers, 9.5 percent self-reported healthcare provider diagnosed lactation mastitis at least once. The strongest risk factors were history of mastitis with a previous child, cracks and nipple sores in the same week, using an antifungal nipple cream (presumably for nipple thrush) in the same week, feeding the baby more frequently, and, for women with no prior mastitis history, using a manual breast pump in the same week. Expressing by hand or pump and hurried or infrequent feeding patterns were thought to be practices associated with mastitis in qualitative interviews of 56 mothers (Potter, 2005). It is unclear if mothers misused the pump, used the pump due to engorgement or other type of milk stasis, or used the pump for any other condition that could contribute to mastitis. This does not appear to be a cause and effect outcome, but more of an association.

Breastmilk and expressed breastmilk are not sterile and can contain a combination of nonpathogenic bacteria and potentially pathogenic species. While full term infants can tolerate higher levels of nonpathogenic bacteria than preterm infants, it is still wise to assure that efforts be made to minimize bacterial contaminants in expressed milk. Heightened awareness in the late 1970s and 1980s regarding the importance of breastmilk for both term and preterm infants was reflected in increased scrutiny of the bacteriologic content of expressed mother's milk (Meier & Wilks, 1987) and efforts were made to reduce bacterial contamination by providing mothers with instructions on how to express milk with low bacteria concentrations (Wilks & Meier, 1988). Contamination of expressed breastmilk could make it unacceptable for feeding to preterm or ill infants (Carroll, Osman, Davies, & McNeish, 1979; Eidelman & Szilagyi, 1979).

Improperly cleaned breast pumps and collection kits can be sources of pathogenic bacteria entering pumped breastmilk (as can unwashed hands or fingers touching any surface that comes into contact with the milk). A number of older studies reported milk contamination traced to or associated with the use of a breast pump (Thom, Cole, & Watrasiewicz, 1970; Pittard, Geddes, Brown, Mintz, & Hulsey, 1991; Boo, Nordiah, Alfizah, & Nor-Rohaini, 2001). Chemical disinfection of older pumps was common, as heat disinfection for non-metal parts was not recommended by manufacturers at that time. Numerous reports mention problems with using a hypochlorite solution to disinfect pump parts. Some of these pumps and cleansing techniques are not currently in use. Pumps have also changed in design to help minimize the chance that bacteria could pass beyond the collection kit and down tubing or into the pump.

Donowitz, Marsik, Fisher, & Wenzel, 1981. Two species of *Klebsiella* bacteria were isolated from a multi-user Egnell electric breast pump in a neonatal intensive care unit (NICU). The pump tubing and overflow bottle safety trap were grossly contaminated with *K. pneumoniae*. A cleansing protocol was instituted for ethylene oxide sterilization of the collection bottle, flange, and tubing that connected to the overflow bottle.

Tyson, Edwards, Rosenfeld, & Beer, 1982. Contaminated milk was observed from the use of Loyd B hand pumps and Egnell electric pumps. Mothers who used Netsy cups (breast shells) had milk that was associated with the highest percentage of contaminated milk pools. Manually expressed milk was less often seen to be contaminated than milk that had been mechanically expressed. Gas autoclaving of contaminated pumps reduced bacterial contamination.

Asquith, Sharp, & Stevenson, 1985. Eighty-five milk samples from 25 mothers using a Medela electric breast pump and 142 milk samples from mothers using a Medela hand pump were collected. The hand pump was also studied with or without applying 1% sodium hypochlorite (household bleach), and air-drying after each use. Results showed that breastmilk with low bacterial counts could be collected with both types of pumps and a collection technique that discarded the first 10 mL of milk expressed. Use of the hypochlorite solution did not provide better disinfection than soap and water washing. They concluded that a simple and adequate cleansing technique of collection kits was to boil all plastic parts for 10 minutes. For disposable kits, washing with hot soapy water, rinsing with fresh water, air-drying, and wrapping in a clean cloth were adequate for same-day use.

Gransden, Webster, French, & Phillips, 1986. Faulty disinfection techniques revealed *Serratia marcescens* in Kaneson hand pumps and an Egnell electric pump. The manual pumps were not completely dismantled before washing and milk was observed under a rubber gasket after washing. Electric pump parts were not fully immersed in the hypochlorite disinfection solution. The solution itself was also seen to be contaminated.

Moloney, Quoraishi, Parry, & Hall, 1987. Serratia marcescens was isolated in a number of multi-user electric pumps (Axicare, Medap, Lothian, Egnell), as well as in hand pumps (Kaneson, Omega) used in the community. Disinfection consisted of washing pump parts with warm water and detergent, then immersing them in a hypochlorite solution. Multiple areas of contamination were found on some of the pumps, especially ones that used overflow bottles.

Blenkharn, 1989. In an experiment on pump contamination, infant formula seeded with *Staphylococcus epidermidis* as the indicator bacteria was seen to pass beyond the collecting bottles of three electric breast pumps (Lactovac Junior, Lactovac Deluxe, and Egnell Lact E). Bacteria were isolated within the first 4–5 cm of the connecting tube between the suction source and the collection bottle, as well as in more distant sites.

Thompson, Pickler, Munro, & Shotwell, 1997. These authors conducted a study to determine if washing the breast with Phisoderm and cleaning the pump flanges immediately before taking a sample of pumped milk resulted in less contamination of the expressed milk. What was noteworthy in the study is that mothers were instructed to wash their pumps parts only once daily with dishwashing detergent. The study showed that the experimental cleansing regimen did not render the expressed milk free of pathogenic bacteria. It is easy to speculate that the improper cleaning instructions could have contributed to such an outcome.

Manufacturer and User Facility Device Experience Database (MAUDE) 1999 (Brown, Bright, Dwyer, & Foxman, 2005). This report refers to a manual breast pump used by a mother of premature twins while they were in the NICU. After the twins became ill, *Pseudomonas aeruginosa* was isolated from the mother's breast pump as the cause of their illness. The mother reported that the tubing from her breast pump system always seemed to have liquid in it. She wondered if this could be the source. The tubing, flange, and valve from the kit, in addition to her pumped breast milk, all grew *P aeruginosa*.

Atkinson, 2001. Cleansing protocols for breast pumps were examined and changed from the use of a hypochlorite solution to the thorough washing, drying, and covering of pump parts. The hypochlorite solution used at that time disinfected, but did not sterilize. The presence of organic matter in the solution inactivated it.

D'Amico, DiNardo, & Krystofiak, 2003. Two breast pump kits used by mothers pumping for preterm infants were cultured in three areas and were positive for *coagulase-negative staphylococci* and *Proteus* species. Cleansing recommendations remained in place to wash the kits in hot soapy water, rinse well, and dry with a paper towel rather than a cloth towel. The kits could also be air dried on a paper towel, but with the parts inverted to drain the water. This was to assure that no bacteria grew in the remaining droplets of water, as *Proteus* had been cultured from the bottom of one of the collection bottles. The cleaned kits were to be covered with a paper towel and left at the bedside of the infant.

Faro, Katz, Berens, & Ross, 2011. A mother presented for her six-week postpartum visit and noted pink discoloration of her First Years breast pump tubing and flanges. *Serratia marcescens* was isolated from both her expressed breast milk and the breast pump. This particular bacterium produces a characteristic brightly colored pink pigment called prodigiosin. The discoloration was noted at the junctions of where one part fit into another. The mother routinely washed the pump equipment between feedings with warm soapy water and microwaved the pump weekly. Based on where the bacterial growth was evident, the pump may not have been completely disassembled when it was cleaned, allowing bacteria to accumulate at the junctures where parts connected to each other.

There is no single evidence-based best method of cleansing or decontaminating breast pumps and their collection kits. Long, complicated, or difficult techniques may result in mothers not cleaning pumps effectively. Thorough washing in hot soapy water to remove all traces of milk, rinsing well, drying, and storing equipment dry in a lightly covered container (so air can circulate and evaporate any remaining moisture) or on dry paper towels seems to yield the best results relative to lowered bacterial concentrations (Gilks, Gould, & Price, 2007). Sterilizing or disinfecting pump parts can be accomplished by boiling the parts, use of an electric sterilizer, placing the parts in a sterilizer bag made for the microwave, or using a dishwasher with a high temperature sanitizing cycle. Cloth towels should be avoided when either drying or storing pump parts. Harsh chemicals and abrasive scrubbing should not be used, as this can create small scratches that can harbor bacteria or mold. Mothers who share an electric pump, such as in a NICU or workplace, should wipe the outside of the pump with a germicidal solution prior to each use. Each step in the breastmilk collection process has the potential to contaminate the milk. It is obviously important that mothers should be instructed in the safest way to collect milk, including how best to clean their pumping equipment (Cossey, Jeurissen, Thelissen, Vanhole, & Schuermans, 2011). Employed mothers who are using electric pumps sometimes have two or three collection kits that they use during their time at work, so they do not need to clean their equipment until they return home. For time strapped mothers in the work setting, some clinicians have recommended that the mothers place their collection kits in a plastic bag in a refrigerator between pumping sessions, rather than taking the time to thoroughly wash all of the parts after pumping. The rationale being that breastmilk is bactericidal and would reduce the chance of high bacterial counts being present during refrigeration. This practice has never been studied for safety and should not be recommended for preterm or ill infants. There is no data on the safety or advisability of this practice. Pump parts can be microwaved between uses in microwave bags that are specifically designed for this use.

Open & Closed Systems

Breast pumps and collection kits for electric breast pumps come in an amazing variety of shapes, sizes, and designs. An important issue to consider when helping mothers determine the correct pump for their needs is whether the pumping system is an open or closed one. A closed collection system has a physical barrier between where the milk enters the collection container and the tubing or part of the pump that leads to the motor (Figure 3.1).

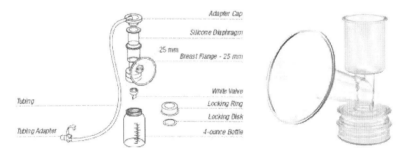

Figure 3.1. A Closed Collection System With a Diaphragm Barrier Between the Air and the Milk.

Source: Ameda pump instruction booklet

The barrier varies among the different pumps and may be a diaphragm or a filter that is impermeable to milk being drawn into the pumping mechanism. In this manner, the milk can never touch the working parts of the pump. This is an important feature to consider if a mother is to use a pump that has been used by other mothers, such as a rental pump or a pump shared by other mothers in a hospital or work setting.

In an open system, there is no physical barrier between where the milk enters the flange and the pump's motor. If expressed milk is not separated from the pump unit by a physical barrier, milk can be drawn back through tubing or the flange directly into the motor each time the motor generates vacuum. This creates a vector for mold, bacteria, and viruses to enter the pump where it is impossible to sterilize. This presents an avenue of contamination for the milk of the mother using the pump, as well as for the milk of the next mother who might use the pump.

Some electric pumping systems have a tendency for moisture to collect in the tubing that runs from the collection kit to the pump. In such a system, if the moisture is not dried after each use, mold can grow in the tubing and contaminate the milk. This is also a sign that milk may have been drawn into the motor itself. So even if a cleaned or new collection kit is used by the mother or the next mother to use the pump, the expressed milk is still at risk of being exposed to the mold and whatever else has been drawn into the pump's motor. Some collection kit designs position the inlets where the milk enters the flange and the inlet where the tubing enters the bottle quite close together, without a physical barrier in between (Figure 3.2). This is an open system. It increases the risk that milk and airflow into the pump can mix freely.

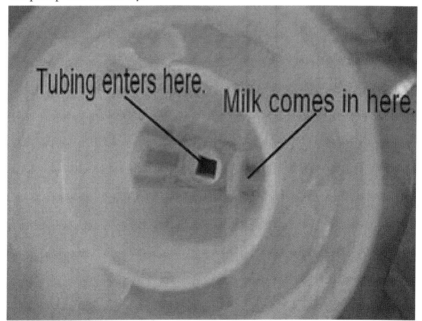

Figure 3.2. Open System Collection Kit

Source: http://mythnomore.blogspot.com/2011/08/why-you-shouldnt-buy-sell-or-borrow.html

No matter how well the outside of the pump is cleaned, the inside of the pump is highly unlikely to have ever been cleaned, making the sharing of open system pumps a poor practice. For example, the Medela Swing pump provides instructions to pump soapy water through the pump itself if there is an overflow of milk. While this cleans the pump, it does not sterilize it or eliminate all potential bacteria or other microbes that may be present.[13]

Mothers can be advised to address moisture in the pump tubing as follows:

- After pumping, remove tubing from the flanges and allow the pump to run for 1–2 minutes until tubing is completely dry.

- Inspect the tubing after each pumping session for condensation and/or milk. If milk appears in tubing:

  ▷ Turn off the pump and unplug from the power source.

  ▷ Remove and disassemble the collection kit and any parts of the pump that the milk has touched. Wash in soapy water, then rinse in clear cold water.

  ▷ Shake water droplets out of the tubing or swing the tubing around your head like a lasso.

  ▷ Hang vertically to air-dry, so that no moisture collects in any curves of the tubing.

- Using an eyedropper, pour a small amount of isopropyl alcohol through the tubing to dry it out and reduce the likelihood of contamination.

- Tubing needs to be replaced if mold is found growing in it, especially if pumping for a preterm or ill infant.

- Tubing can be boiled, but this may cause it to become opaque, making it more difficult to see condensation or milk droplets if present.

Sharing a Pump or Buying a Used Pump

Many mothers wish to save money on breast pump equipment and may gratefully accept a pump previously used by another mother. Other mothers may wish to purchase a used breast pump to reduce the strain on

---

13 http://mythnomore.blogspot.com/2011/08/why-you-shouldnt-buy-sell-or-borrow.html

the family budget. The FDA discourages this practice and provides a clear warning regarding sharing pumps or purchasing a used pump (Box 3.4).[14]

Box 3.4. The FDA's Position on Shared and Used Breast Pumps

Should I Buy a Used Breast Pump or Share a Breast Pump?

You should never buy a used breast pump or share a breast pump.

Only FDA cleared hospital-grade pumps should be used by more than one person. With the exception of hospital-grade pumps, the FDA considers breast pumps single-use devices. This means that a breast pump should only be used by one woman because there is no way to guarantee the pump can be cleaned and disinfected between uses by different women.

The money you may save by buying a used pump is not worth the health risks to you or your baby. Breast pumps that are reused by different mothers can carry infectious diseases, such as HIV or hepatitis.

Buying a used breast pump or sharing a breast pump may be a violation of the manufacturer's warranty, and you may not be able to get help from the manufacturer if you have a problem with the pump.

Source: http://www.fda.gov/MedicalDevices/ProductsandMedicalProcedures/ HomeHealthandConsumer/ConsumerProducts/BreastPumps/ucm061939.htm

Many breast pump companies are sufficiently concerned about this practice that they will not sell collection kits and replacement parts for used personal-use pumps. Manufacturer's generally discourage sharing or purchasing used breast pumps, not to increase profits, but because many pumps cannot be sterilized between users and may wear out (Box 3.5).

---

14 http://www.fda.gov/MedicalDevices/ProductsandMedicalProcedures/ HomeHealthandConsumer/ConsumerProducts/BreastPumps/ucm061939.htm

Box 3.5. Medela Inc.'s Warning on the Sharing or Using of Pre-Owned Breast Pumps[15]

Many mothers have asked if they can safely sell, purchase, or use a previously owned breast pump. Medela is concerned about the health and welfare of breastfeeding mothers and their babies. There is evidence that bacteria and certain viruses may be transmittable through breastmilk. For this reason, it is not advisable to use a previously owned, personal-use breast pump, such as *Medela's Pump In Style*. However, it is safe to use a Rental pump, such as *Medela's Symphony* or *Lactina* pumps. The difference between personal-use pumps and rental pumps is as follows:

Personal-Use Breast pumps

Personal-use pumps that you buy at the store are personal-care items, much like a toothbrush. Personal-use pumps should never be resold or shared among mothers. The *Medela Pump In Style Advanced* has an internal diaphragm that cannot be removed, replaced, or fully sterilized. Therefore, the risk of cross-contamination associated with re-using a previously owned pump, such as the Pump In Style, cannot be dismissed, even when using a new kit or tubing. Similarly, the *Medela Single Deluxe* breast pump has an internal motor that cannot be removed, replaced, or fully sterilized. Another consideration when deciding to borrow or even lend a previously owned electric pump is the pump's motor life. A high quality electric double pump might last through the breastfeeding of your second child, or even several children. However, like computers or other electronic products, an electric breast pump has a limited lifetime. Medela guarantees its pump motors with a one-year warranty. If you use an electronic pump that has been used for more than one year, there is no guarantee that it will generate as much speed and vacuum as it did earlier in it's life. By using your own pump, you can compare the pump's performance with each child. However, if you borrow a pump, you cannot gauge its performance to ensure it is operating at full capacity.

Rental Pumps

Rental pumps, such as *Medela's Symphony* and *Lactina,* are designed for multiple users. These pumps have special barriers and filters to prohibit milk from entering the pump motor, which prevent cross-contamination. In addition, each renter uses her own personal set of breastshields, containers, and tubing to ensure the safe use of these pumps.

Source: http://www.medelabreastfeedingus.com/tips-and-solutions/14/can-i-buy-or-borrow-a-pre-owned-breastpump

---

15 http://www.medelabreastfeedingus.com/tips-and-solutions/14/can-i-buy-or-borrow-a-pre-owned-breastpump

On a Medela Pump In Style breast pump, the rubber diaphragm that creates the vacuum can be contaminated by moisture or milk that enters through the tubing. Mothers can remove the faceplate on this pump, inspect it, and let it dry. The diaphragm itself cannot be sterilized. While this is a popular pump, clinicians can explain to mothers why it should not be used by more than one mother.

Use of a shared pump or purchase of a used pump invalidates the manufacturer's warranty, meaning there will be no recourse from the manufacturer if the pump breaks or fails. These warranties are often valid for only one year, with some of the smaller pumps and hand-helds having warranties that last a mere 90 days. In addition to concerns regarding pump contamination, used pumps come with another set of problems related to their longevity. The motors in these pumps have a limited lifetime, sometimes just long enough for pumping for one baby. Over time, especially with heavy use, pump motors may start to be less effective. Their suction may diminish or their cycling patterns may change. This means that a mother who pumps with a used breast pump may put her milk supply at risk with a pump that is not working well enough to stimulate continued good milk production. The pump may have been heavily used already, lowering the life expectancy of the motor. This becomes more serious if a mother is dependent on this pump for continued milk production because she is employed full time or is pumping for a preterm or ill infant. A mother may not realize that her borrowed or used pump is not working correctly, and it is this factor that could be responsible for her diminishing milk production. Used pumps may break, necessitating the purchase of another pump. If the pump was borrowed, there may be a perceived obligation to replace it, costing the mother more money than if she purchased a new one. Purchasing a used breast pump online or one that is claimed to be new and unused places the buyer in a precarious position. There is no way to know how long or how heavily the pump has been used, nor is there any way to know if the internal mechanisms have been contaminated by milk, bacteria, viruses, yeast, or mold. While a clinician can use a pressure gauge to determine if the pump's vacuum is performing to specifications, there is no algorithm to allow the health professional to gauge how much life is left in the pump or how much longer it will work in the way it was intended.

Cost of Breast Pumps

Many mothers are concerned about the cost of either purchasing or renting a breast pump. Pump costs range from approximately $18 for a manual pump to more than $1200 for a large hospital-grade multi-user pump. Sometimes it helps mothers put in perspective what their financial investment in a breast pump means to themselves and their family (Figure 3.3).

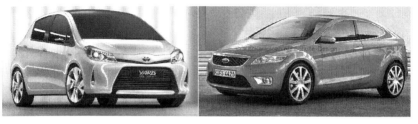

Toyota Yaris $271/mo = $3252/year   Ford Focus $279/mo = $3348/year

Figure 3.3. Cost of Powdered Formula for One Year Compared to Cost of Car Payments for One Year

The cost of one year of powdered formula can be almost as much as five car payments. Large electric breast pumps can be rented and are a good option for employed mothers and a necessity for mothers of preterm infants. Rental rates vary by area of the country and type of pump that is rented. Rental rates for a hospital-grade multi-user pump can run from $50 to $80 per month. Renting for multiple months lowers the cost even more. The double collection kit costs between $46 and $56. Popular personal-use pumps range from over $100 to over $300 and may be out of the financial reach of some mothers, especially if they are returning to employment after their maternity leave. The cost to rent a pump or purchase a personal-use pump is still less, however, than missing days from work or purchasing infant formula. Mothers enrolled in the Special Supplemental Nutrition Program for Women, Infants, and Children (WIC) may be able to secure, borrow, or rent pumps from their local WIC office. In 1989, Congress authorized states to purchase breast pumps with Nutrition Services Administration funds.[16] In 1998, Congress authorized the use of WIC food funds to purchase breast pumps.[17] These two funding options made it possible for all state agencies to provide breast pumps to participants. States have the option of giving single-user pumps to mothers or selling them to mothers at a nominal cost. States may also loan or rent multi-user pumps or contract with a third party to provide pumps to participants. Third parties may include lactation consultants, hospitals, or durable medical equipment (DME) vendors. Medicaid programs should be contacted to determine whether and under what circumstances Medicaid will provide

---

16 The Child Nutrition and WIC Reauthorization Act of 1989 (Public Law 101-147)
17 The William F. Goodling Child Nutrition Reauthorization Act of 1998 (Public Law 105-336)

pumps for medical necessity to WIC mothers.[18] Sometimes, however, loaner breast pumps are in short supply in WIC offices and demand simply exceeds supply.

Some mothers might be fortunate enough to take advantage of hospital programs that give, loan, or rent pumps at low cost, such as the Pumps for Peanuts program at Boston Medical Center (Philipp, Brown, & Merewood, 2000). The program guarantees that every NICU mother has access to a double-electric pump, regardless of health insurance or financial status. A standing physician's order ensures that every NICU mother, if she chooses to breastfeed, is offered a hospital-owned electric breast pump immediately after her infant is born. Funding for the program comes from a grant from the hospital's charity foundation.

Accessing appropriate electric breast pumps for use by inner city, low-income mothers with ill or preterm infants or impoverished mothers who must return to work within a few weeks of delivery can be quite daunting. Chamberlain, McMahon, Philipp, & Merewood (2006) identified a number of challenges that inner city mothers encounter when attempting to secure an electric breast pump:

- Even if they have insurance coverage for a breast pump, mothers have difficulty accessing a pump because local pharmacies in the inner city frequently do not accept insurance reimbursements for breast pumps.

- Some pharmacies will provide a mother with an unsuitable pump, such as a "bicycle horn" hand pump, rather than a multi-user hospital-grade electric pump.

Some pharmacies, pump depots, or DME vendors do not accept Medicaid insurance plans. Providers of breast pumps often must deal with mothers who are transient, lack transportation, may not speak English, and do not return the rental pumps. This further limits pump availability. In an attempt to improve access to breast pumps for all breastfeeding mothers who needed one, a Boston, Massachusetts, inner city hospital worked with local insurers and breast pump distributors to arrange for pump access for their insured patients (Chamberlain et al., 2006). The Breastfeeding Center at the hospital negotiated the provision of pumps by a number of insurers whereby a personal-use breast pump was given to insured mothers. This proved to be such a popular benefit that many women actually switched their insurance coverage plans to one that covered breast pumps. Many insurers came on board with this arrangement because they actually gained

---

18 http://www.paramountcommunication.com/nwica/
GuidelinesforWICAgenciesProvidingBreastPumps.pdf

clientele through this program. The question arose that the type of pump being provided may not be the optimal pump for all situations. While clinical experience points to the recommendation that mothers of preterm or ill infants typically use a hospital-grade multi-user double electric pump, the personal-use pump was deemed better than no pump at all, which had been the norm. The personal-use pump was chosen to be given to mothers because the breast pump distributors had lost excessive amounts of money with hospital-grade rental pumps that were never returned, and they no longer offered the rental pump option.

Insurance Coverage for Breast Pumps

Insurance coverage for breast pumps has varied widely, from some insurers covering no breast pumps for any reason to others paying for rental breast pumps as long as the infant is hospitalized. Coverage has been uneven and spotty, with some mothers required to provide co-pays or pay the amount that exceeds caps placed on the maximum the insurer intends to pay for a pump. Some mothers have wondered why an insurer who pays for breast pumps will not pay for a pump in their particular situation. This may occur when an employer is self-insured. This means that the employer is actually the insurer and simply contracts with an insurance company to administer employee claims. Employers can "carve out" what they do not wish to pay for, and often breast pumps are denied for reimbursement because of this option.

However, in March of 2010, the Affordable Care Act (ACA)—the health insurance reform legislation passed by Congress, was signed into law by President Obama. This is designed to make preventive services and equipment affordable and accessible for all Americans by requiring health plans to cover preventive services and by eliminating cost sharing.[19] In addition, in July 2011, the Institute of Medicine (IOM) issued guidelines with respect to the preventive services for **women** for purposes of implementing the ACA. These recommendations, which have been endorsed by the Department of Health and Human Services (HHS), include coverage for "lactation counseling and equipment to help women who choose to breastfeed to do so successfully."[20] Under the ACA, health insurers will be required to pay for a range of preventative care services specifically aimed at women. Required health plan coverage guidelines specify that non-grandfathered plans and issuers are required to provide

19   U.S. Preventive Services Task Force, Primary Care Preventions to Promote Breastfeeding, http://www.uspreventiveservicestaskforce.org/uspstf/uspsbrfd.htm.

20   Institute of Medicine, Clinical Preventive Services for Women: Closing the Gaps (July 2011), available at http://www.iom.edu/Reports/2011/Clinical-Preventive-Services-for-Women-Closing-the-Gaps.aspx.

coverage without cost sharing, consistent with these guidelines in the first plan year (in the individual market, policy year) that begins on or after August 1, 2012.[21] These requirements include:

- Breastfeeding support, supplies, and counseling.

- Comprehensive lactation support and counseling, by a trained provider during pregnancy and/or in the postpartum period, and costs for renting breastfeeding equipment.

While this is not a perfect system for breast pump coverage as it does not apply to all health plans, many mothers will soon be able to take advantage of improved access to the equipment that they need. Clinicians and mothers will need to be aware of which health plans are required to provide coverage for breast pumps. Any time a mother is denied health insurance coverage for breast pumps needed for a medical indication, it should first be appealed to the insurer. If the appeal process fails, then the lack of coverage should be reported to the state insurance commissioner's office. States have an on-line complaint form that both clinicians and mothers can submit when they feel that needed coverage has been denied.

Health insurers are familiar with covering breast pumps and replacement parts, as specific codes exist for these items within the Healthcare Common Procedure Coding System (HCPCS). When medical equipment distributors, pump depots, DMEs, etc. bill an insurer for a breast pump or replacement parts, a specific code is used that tells the insurer what services have been rendered, in this case the provision of a breast pump. A typical code set appears in Box 3.6.

Box 3.6. HCPCS Codes for Breast Pumps and Replacement Parts

A4281 - A4286 Breast pump supplies

E0602 Breast pump, manual, any type

E0603 Breast pump, electric (AC and/or DC), any type

E0604 Breast pump, hospital grade, electric (AC and/or DC), any type

Source: http://www.icd9data.com/HCPCS/2012/E/default.htm and http://www.icd9data.com/HCPCS/2012/A/default.htm

Mothers received a bonus from the Internal Revenue Service (IRS), which now allows breast pumps and supplies that assist lactation to be

---

21 http://www.hrsa.gov/womensguidelines/

deducted as medical expenses on tax returns[22] and to be covered under an employee's flexible health spending account.[23] The IRS reversed its position on breast pumps and lactation equipment in response to a letter sent by legislators explaining the importance of this equipment for continued breastfeeding in certain circumstances. The legislators urged the IRS to allow pumps to be covered under flexible health spending accounts and make them tax deductible on mothers' tax returns (Clinical Lactation, 2011).

22 http://www.irs.gov/pub/irs-pdf/p502.pdf
23 http://www.irs.gov/pub/irs-drop/a-11-14.pdf

Part 2.
The World of Breast Pumps

Chapter 4. Mechanics

The dairy industry is probably the all time expert on pumps and pumping milk! There are some interesting similarities and, of course, many differences between a commercial milking apparatus and a breast pump. The four teats on a dairy cow are milked with a teat cup apparatus that fits snuggly over each teat and alternates applying vacuum and allowing the teat to rest between vacuum applications. A vacuum of 279 mmHg to 304 mmHg is continuously applied with an inner liner in the teat cup, as well as in the area between the inner liner and the steel casing. This is the maximum amount of vacuum to which the tip of the teat is exposed. The rubber liner collapses periodically to massage the teat, but more importantly to close off the vacuum and allow the teat to rest between vacuum applications (Figure 4.1). This alternating application of vacuum and rest occurs at 60 cycles per minute. A typical cycling ratio of 60/40 applies vacuum for 60% of each cycle and interrupts vacuum or allows a rest period for 40% of the cycle. The milking apparatus can milk the front two teats at a different rate than the hind two teats, as the back of the udder tends to have more milk. Modern dairies can use a computerized system that programs how the udder will be milked and measures the milk output of each cow. Cows are generally milked twice a day.

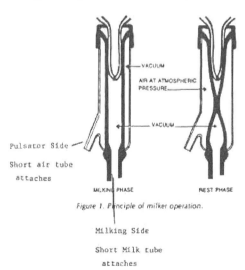

Figure 1. Principle of milker operation.

Figure 4.1. Teat Cup Showing Inner Liner Open and Closed

Source: http://cal.vet.upenn.edu/projects/fieldservice/Dairy/Mastitis/milkmac.htm

Breast pumps also provide vacuum and rest cycles and have cycling ratios, but few have a collapsible-type flange. There are three basic types of breast pumps based on how vacuum is generated—hand pumps that generate vacuum by squeezing or operating a handle, battery-operated pumps with small motors whose power is supplied by batteries, and electrically operated pumps. Pump mechanisms are usually either a piston arrangement, where a piston is drawn through a cylinder to create suction, or a diaphragm arrangement, where a diaphragm is pulled or pulsates to provide vacuum. Clinicians interested in learning about the specifications, drawings, claims, and narratives for how a particular pump works can access the website of the United States Patent and Trademark Office at http://www.uspto.gov/index.jsp and look up the pump in which they are interested. For example, the Symphony breast pump from Medela Inc. has 23 pages devoted to its patent, which was granted in 2003 (Figure 4.2). Also included in the patent specifications were examples of the suction curves generated by the pump, as well as the cycles per minute and the amount of vacuum that the pump generated (Figure 4.3). Revisions to pumps and changes in pumps are an ongoing process and happen quite frequently.

U.S. Patent   Apr. 15, 2003   Sheet 13 of 15   US 6,547,756 B1

FIG. 22

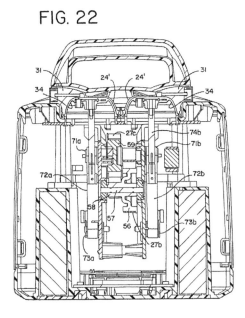

Figure 4.2. Sample of Internal Specifications in the Patent of the Symphony Pump Taken From Its Patent Application

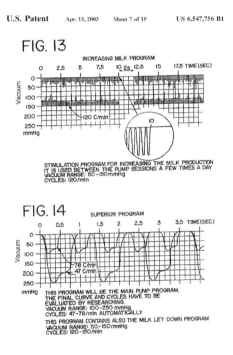

Figure 4.3. Differing Suction Curves Within the Programmable Symphony Pump Taken From Its Patent Application

Vacuum

The vacuum applied to the breast by an infant during suckling is not constant. The infant grasps the nipple/areola and initiates vacuum to draw the nipple/areolar complex into his mouth. Vacuum rises as the nipple/areolar complex is drawn further into the mouth. Vacuum is interrupted during swallowing, but not completely released, as some vacuum needs to be exerted as a basal resting pressure to keep the nipple in the mouth. The vacuum stretches the nipple/areolar complex to approximately twice its resting length, with a 70 percent reduction of the teat's original diameter (Smith, Erenberg, & Nowak, 1988; Weber, Woolridge, & Baum, 1986). Authors have speculated on the function of vacuum during sucking, with thoughts that (1) vacuum facilitates the refilling of the ducts with milk within the nipple following each swallow or (2) milk is released from the nipple by vacuum caused when the jaw lowers and enlarges the oral cavity (Smith et al., 1988). In a breastfeeding ultrasound study, Jacobs, Dickinson, Hart, Doherty, and Faulkner (2007) stated that the tongue in its most elevated position secured the nipple in contact with the hard palate, but did not compress any milk into the oral cavity. Tongue movement downward was followed by milk exiting the nipple. Other ultrasound studies showed that when the posterior part of the tongue was lowered during sucking at the breast, milk ducts in the nipple opened and milk flowed into the infant's mouth. When the tongue was raised, neither milk ducts in the nipple nor milk flow were observed. Milk appeared to be captured in the nipple, ready to flow into the infant's mouth when the jaw was lowered again, but peristaltic tongue movements did not seem to be observed (Geddes, Kent, Mitoulas, & Hartmann, 2008). The tongue was described as moving up and down, creating vacuum in the baby's palate in front of the nipple and inducing milk flow. Woolridge (2011), in ultrasound studies of breastfeeding infants, found that vacuum was not the only force involved in extracting milk, but that peristaltic motions of the tongue were visible. He determined that vacuum and peristaltic motions of the tongue (compressive forces or positive pressure) worked synergistically to extract milk. Monaci & Woolridge (2011) reported that in ultrasound imaging of infants suckling at the breast, the tongue was seen to change configuration—during peristaltic action (positive pressure or compressive action), the tongue moved in a peristaltic wave, and during vacuum action, the tongue moved up and down with a flatter profile. An infant feeding at breast demonstrates 42 to 126 suck cycles per minute, with a mean of 74 sucks per minute (Bowen-Jones, Thompson, & Drewett, 1982). Suction is thought to be applied over approximately half of the suck cycle (Halverson, 1944). Lower vacuums may be best used for mothers with sore nipples or engorgement, while higher vacuums may be better for mothers who are pump dependent or employed mothers who must empty the breast as thoroughly as possible to maintain good milk production.

Cycles Per Minute

Cycles per minute refers to the number of times each minute the pump can increase vacuum, reach peak vacuum, and release vacuum. Pumps with low cycling are generally not as effective as those with higher cycling capability. A pump that can establish at least 40 to 60 cycles per minute generally results in better milk yields, especially if mothers are using the pump on a daily basis (Alekseev, Omel'ianuk, & Talalaeva, 2000). Pumps that generate less than this number of cycles per minute are more appropriate for occasional pumping.

Suction Curves

A suction curve is a graphic representation of how fast and high suction is generated, when and if it is released, and how rapidly it falls before the next vacuum cycle is generated (Figure 4.3). Suction curves in an electric pump vary from pump to pump and manufacturer to manufacturer. For example, one type of suction curve may have a rapid generation of suction and another may have a smooth suction curve, with a slight hold at the maximum vacuum. Some curves have a quick vacuum release. The Ameda electric pumps have a short push, with positive pressure at the end of each cycle that allows the nipple to re-perfuse with blood and milk. The bottom line of Figure 4.4 is the vacuum curve for the Simplisse electric pump.

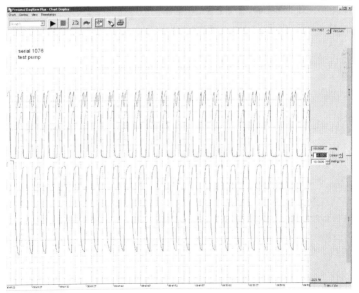

Figure 4.4. Vacuum Curve (Bottom Line) for the Simplisse Electric Pump

Source: Simplisse.

Vacuum in a breast pump is generated in differing manners, depending on the type of pump. Most pumps have a range of vacuum that can be generated, generally as a preset function. Vacuum or suction is not the only force that an infant employs to extract milk from the breast.

Compression

A compressive force from the infant's tongue and jaw is also applied to capture milk within the nipple, and if peristaltic actions of the tongue occur, to assist in milk movement through the nipple. The compressive force in a breast pump would come from contact made between the nipple/areola that has been drawn into the nipple tunnel of the flange. The nipple/areola is compressed against a hard plastic flange surface, or in a few breast pumps, against flanges that have a soft inner liner that pulsates against the nipple/areola.

Studies were conducted that used computer modeling to compare breastfeeding and breast pumps. There seems to be an optimal time during the suction cycle when an infant applies the compressive peristaltic force of the tongue. This results in an asymmetric compression of the nipple/areola between the tongue and hard palate. Using a model that applied symmetric peristaltic compression of a "nipple" during a suction cycle, Zoppou, Barry, & Mercer (1997[a]) found that the compressive force applied at the optimal time and speed during the suck cycle could significantly increase the mean fluid flow through the teat, while a compressive force applied at the wrong time in the pressure cycle restricted the flow of fluid. A compressive force applied by a breast pump approximately a quarter of the way through the suction cycle increased the milk volume over one suction cycle by 15 percent, while a compressive force that compressed the teat early in the suction cycle restricted milk flow into the teat and reduced the theoretical milk volume (Zoppou, Barry, & Mercer, 1997b). Alekseev and colleagues (1998) found that adding the compressive stimulus to a breast pump changed the dynamics of milk expression. Using an experimental pump where the compressive stimulus could be switched on and off, it was found that in a three to five minute period of pumping, 50 percent of the milk could be removed from the breast, but when the compressive stimulus was turned off, it took 1.5 to 2.0 times longer to express this volume of milk.

Several breast pumps over the years have included flanges that are designed to apply positive pressure to the breast. In an attempt to create a breast pump that provided both positive and negative pressure, Whittlestone (1978) devised a breast pump that employed simultaneous pumping of both breasts and adopted principles from the commercial dairy milking machines. The flanges of the Whittlestone pump provided a compressive force to the breast from a liner inside the pump flange that rhythmically contracted around the nipple/areola. He called this a physiologic breastmilker. Its gentle vacuum did not cycle, but the flange liners contracted rhythmically to interrupt the vacuum. The pump was anecdotally reported as being insufficient for many mothers, as it did not seem to pump as much milk as other double-electric pumps. Only one paper could be located on this pump which stated it was effective for helping relieve engorgement.[24] It is no longer on the market (Figure 4.5).

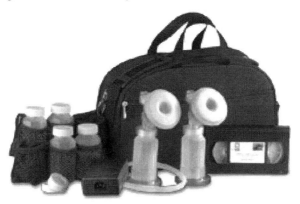

Figure 4.5. Whittlestone Breast Expresser With Pulsating Inner Flange Liner

The Whisper Wear breast pump (Figure 4.6) was designed to be a hands-free pump worn under each bra cup, which utilized a flexible massaging liner that enveloped the nipple and areola. It was battery operated and the milk drained down a tube into a collecting bag. Many mothers found this pump to be very convenient, but anecdotal reports mentioned that sometimes the fit between the flange and the breast was not good. The pump had only one size. Some mothers complained that the vacuum was insufficient for their needs or that their nipple/areola did not fit well within the nipple tunnel. The Whisper Wear pump is no longer on the market.

---

24 http://www.whittlestone.com/documents/breastengorgementtreatment.pdf

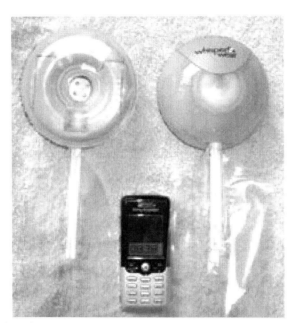

Figure 4.6. The Whisper Wear Pump Worn Under Each Bra Cup

Other pumps have a soft flange that collapse over the teat when vacuum is applied. The flanges of the Simplisse breast pump have an inner liner that pulsates and provides limited compression over the breast (Figure 4.7).

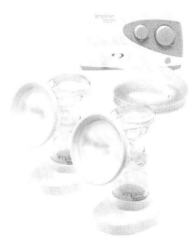

Figure 4.7. The Simplisse Flanges Pulsate Over the Breast Providing Gentle Compression

Hormonal Issues

A breast pump expressing breastmilk is not the same as an infant feeding at the breast. Breast pumps are not as efficient as an infant in removing milk from the breasts. Breast pumps must act on the breast, neurological system, and endocrine system in a manner that will promote the release of prolactin and oxytocin and drain the breasts sufficiently to signal the need for continued milk synthesis. Prolactin and oxytocin are the main hormones of importance in initiating and sustaining milk production. The characteristics of breast pumps must be able to positively influence release of these hormones in order for mothers to initiate and sustain milk production on a short- and long-term basis.

Prolactin

Prolactin levels rise steadily during pregnancy to prepare the breasts for lactation (Neville, 1983). Prolactin levels increase from about 10 ng/ml in the nonpregnant state to approximately 200 ng/ml at term. Baseline levels during lactation remain somewhat elevated and average approximately 100 ng/ml at three months and 50 ng/ml at six months. Prolactin levels, however, rise dramatically under the sucking stimulus of an infant to about double, with suckling being the most powerful natural stimulus for prolactin release. After about six months of breastfeeding, the prolactin rise with suckling amounts to only about 5 to 10 ng/ml. This is thought to occur due to the increased prolactin binding capacity or sensitivity of the mammary tissue that allows full lactation in the face of falling prolactin levels over time. The high levels of prolactin during pregnancy and early lactation contribute to the increase in the number of prolactin receptors within the breast and are dependant on tactile input for stimulation and release. Prolactin does not directly regulate the short-term or long-term rate of milk synthesis (Cox, Owens, & Hartmann, 1996). Prolactin is particularly important for the initiation of milk production, but once lactation is well established, prolactin, while still required for milk synthesis to occur, assumes its role as permissive rather than regulatory (Cregan & Hartmann, 1999).

Prolactin concentration in the plasma operates as a true circadian rhythm, being highest during sleep and lowest during the waking hours (Stern & Reichlin, 1990). The prolactin response is superimposed on the circadian rhythm of prolactin secretion. This has implications for when the best time might be to pump the highest volume of milk. The stimulus from a breast pump may be able to elevate prolactin levels more effectively during the night when the circadian input enhances the effect of the sucking stimulus (Freeman, Kanyicska, Lerant, & Nagy, 2000). A number of small studies, with wide variations in methodology, have demonstrated the ability of various older pumps to elevate prolactin levels (Noel, Suh, & Frantz, 1974; Weichert, 1980; Howie, McNeilly, McArdle, Smart, Houston, 1980; de Sanctis, Vitali, Atti, Vullo, Sabato, & Bagni, 1981; Neifert & Seacat, 1985; Zinaman et al., 1992). A study that compared preterm pump-dependent mothers with full-term breastfeeding mothers showed that preterm mothers who double pumped with a hospital-grade electric pump had elevated prolactin levels similar to those of term mothers during feeding of their infant at the breast (Hill et al., 2009). This is important, as preterm mothers tend to have lower basal prolactin levels than what is normal for term mothers. In this study there was a significant interaction between prolactin levels and frequency of breast stimulation with a pump.

Encouraging preterm mothers to pump more frequently will expose the breasts to higher than basal levels of prolactin over a longer period of time, which may help increase pumped milk volumes in a situation known for milk production difficulties. In a study that compared the prolactin response to pumping using two different electric breast pumps (Embrace by Playtex and Pump In Style by Medela), it was demonstrated that the prolactin response was greater with the Embrace pump, but milk extraction efficiency was greater with the Pump In Style pump. The pumps did not differ in their ability to increase milk production over time or in their ability to support long-term milk production (Hopkinson & Heird, 2009). The authors discuss how the Embrace pump stimulated the endocrine half of the milk production system and the Pump In Style stimulated the autocrine arm. While the mothers in the study alternately used both pumps during the study period, they were no more likely to choose one pump over the other in terms of which pump they chose to keep. The two pumps seemed comparable for long-term ability to support adequate milk production when using the pump twice per day.

Clinical Implications

1. *The function of infant suckling (or mechanical milk removal) varies between lactogenesis II, the onset of copious milk production, and lactogenesis III, the maintenance of abundant milk production.* Lactogenesis II or the milk coming in, can take place in the absence of milk removal over the first three days postpartum, but milk composition will not mature and milk volume will not increase to maximum milk production in the absence of frequent milk removal after that time. While suckling (or mechanical milk removal) may not be a prerequisite for lactogenesis II, it is critical for lactogenesis III. Delayed suckling by

the infant, whether due to premature delivery (Cregan, DeMello, & Hartmann 2000), cesarean delivery (Sozmen, 1992), or other perinatal factors that would necessitate mechanical milk removal, may affect the timing or delay the onset of lactogenesis II. Delayed onset of lactation can often result in unnecessary formula supplementation, low milk supply, and premature weaning. Additional breast pumping after a couple of breastfeeds *before* the onset of lactogenesis II has not been shown to hasten the event or result in increased milk transfer to the baby at 72 hours (Chapman, Young, Ferris, & Pérez-Escamilla, 2001). In the absence of a baby at breast (such as with a preterm infant or one who is unable to latch), the breasts need to be stimulated eight or more times every 24 hours to assure that the breast is exposed to prolactin and primed for adequate milk production. Pumping only once or twice during the day and never at night, when prolactin levels are at their peak, may contribute to delayed lactogenesis II. A faltering milk supply in the following weeks may be attributed to the lack of sufficient prolactin receptors and infrequent breast stimulation while lactation is being established. The first 14 days set the stage for the volume of milk that will be produced during the current lactation.

2. *Painful overdistention of the breasts (secondary engorgement) must be prevented.* As pressure within the alveolar (milk-secreting) cells rises, suppression of milk synthesis begins. Painful engorgement lasting longer than 48 hours has the potential to decrease the milk supply. Therefore, if a baby cannot keep up with the abrupt increase in milk production, the mother should express her excess milk. When milk production begins in the absence of a baby directly feeding at the breast, pumping frequency may need to be temporarily increased to prevent involution of the alveoli caused by the back pressure of milk and the buildup of suppressor peptides that down-regulate milk volume. Wilde, Prentice, & Peaker (1995) have identified this peptide and named it the feedback inhibitor of lactation (FIL).

3. *The first two weeks of breastfeeding are a critical period of time during which frequent nipple stimulation and milk removal are necessary for an abundant milk supply during the remainder of the lactation.* Management guidelines should include instructions for frequent pumping if the mother and baby are separated or if the infant cannot latch directly to the breast or remove adequate amounts of milk. Woolridge (1995) provided a practical identification of six separate stages in the lactation process:

   ▷ Priming (changes of pregnancy).

▷ Initiation (birth and the management of early breastfeeding).

▷ Calibration (the concept that milk production gets underway without the breasts actually "knowing" how much milk to make in the beginning). Over the first three to five weeks, milk output is progressively calibrated to the baby's needs, usually building up (up-regulation), but occasionally down-regulating to meet the baby's needs.

▷ Maintenance (the period of exclusive breastfeeding).

▷ Decline (the period after complementary foods or supplements are added).

▷ Involution (weaning).

It is the second, third, and fourth time periods that are crucial to ensuring abundant milk production. Mothers who are pump dependent or whose infant is not able to maintain sufficient intake when feeding directly at the breast are at risk of producing insufficient milk unless the breasts are adequately "calibrated" during these periods of time. While milk production can usually be increased later on, it can be much more difficult to catch up the milk production than to calibrate it high to begin with.

Several studies have shown that total expressed milk volume tends to be higher when using a breast pump compared to manual expression. Paul, Singh, Deorari, Pacheco, & Taneja (1996) showed that use of a cylinder pump resulted in significantly higher volumes of milk expressed per session compared to hand expression.

Slusher et al. (2007) compared milk volumes expressed by hand, double collection pedal pump, and double collection electric pump. Each of the pumps resulted in higher expressed milk volumes compared to hand expression, with the double collection electric pump expressing the highest volume of milk among the three methods. However, while there was a significant difference between electric breast pump expression and hand expression, there was not much difference in mean daily expressed milk volume between the electric pump and pedal pump or the pedal pump and hand expression. Another study conducted with three groups of mothers whose infants were too preterm or ill to feed directly at the breast and who were using either a double electric pump, a manual pump, or hand expression found that the use of a double electric pump produced a greater mean volume of breastmilk than hand expression. However, hand expression and the hand pump still yielded sufficient milk for some of the mothers in the study (Slusher et al., 2011). According to Ingram and colleagues (1999), the estimated mean milk volume produced by term mothers by day seven is 576 mL for infants feeding at the breast (range 200 to 1,013 mL). For the three groups in this study, mothers in the electric pump group expressed 647 mL per day, the single non-electric pump group expressed 520 mL of milk per day, and the mothers who were hand expressing yielded 434 mL per day. This has implications for pumping in developing countries where electricity and electric pumps may not be readily available.

While use of a double electric breast pump may produce a greater volume of milk over a longer period of time, an important role for hand expression has been revealed, especially during the first 48 hours (Ohyama, Watabe, & Hayasaka, 2010) and beyond (Morton, 2009). Ohyama, Watabe, & Hayasaka (2010) found that manual expression yielded twice as much colostrum as did electric pumping during the first 48 hours following delivery in mothers who delivered between 29 and 39 weeks. Mothers in this study alternated between manual expression and using a double electric pump such that every other expression session was done by hand. Other studies have shown that improved colostrum yield can be significant and increased milk yields over time have been shown when electric breast pump use and hand expression are combined early after birth (Morton et al., 2009).

Studies have shown that there is a relationship between how thoroughly the breast is drained at each feeding or pumping and the amount of milk that is produced to replace it. It was found that the degree of breast emptying is inversely proportional to the amount of milk subsequently synthesized; that is, the more thoroughly a breast is drained, the more milk is made (Daly et al., 1992; Daly, Owens, & Hartmann, 1993). It has been noted that breasts with smaller storage capacities may need to be expressed more frequently than breasts with larger storage capacities, even though both types of breasts are capable of synthesizing similar amounts of milk in a 24-hour period (Daly & Hartmann, 1995a, 1995b). Mothers with larger storage capacities are able to express a higher volume of milk with each pumping session, but not necessarily more milk in a 24-hour period than mothers with smaller storage capacities. A relationship has been found between the volume of milk that is expressed during a pumping and how full the breast is at that time. The fuller the breast the higher the milk yield (Mitoulas, Lai, & Gurrin, Larson, & Hartmann, 2002b). The fuller the breast the less time it seems to take to achieve the milk-ejection reflex, with a less full breast taking up to 120 seconds (Hartmann, 2002). Mothers may notice that one breast tends to produce more milk than the other. Often, expressed milk volume tends to be higher from the right breast than the left, with these differences sometimes being quite large but stable over time. The differences can appear quite early in lactation and are not related to total milk output (Engstrom, Meier, Jegier, Motykowski, & Zuleger, 2007). Primiparous mothers and mothers breastfeeding for the first time demonstrated the greatest differences. While the exact reason for this difference is not known, a possible explanation could be that the right breast preferentially receives more blood flow than the left, which was demonstrated in a Doppler ultrasound study in women with established lactation (Aljazaf, 2004). Even though differing milk outputs between breasts is normal, the clinician needs to make sure there are no other problems that would account for this discrepancy, such as a plugged duct, mastitis, improperly fitted pump flange that is too tight, any surgical procedures on the breast (a biopsy, nipple piercing, augmentation or reduction surgery), or an anomalous breast that is hypoplastic.

Oxytocin

Oxytocin is the hormone that activates the milk-ejection reflex. Oxytocin acts on the myoepithelial processes, causing shortening of the ducts without constricting them, which increases the milk pressure. Cobo, De Bernal, Gaitan, & Quintero (1967) measured milk-ejection by recording intraductal mammary pressure using a catheter placed in a mammary duct. Ductal pressures went from 0 to 25 mmHg on the recording paper. Ductal contractions lasted about one minute and were measured as occurring about four to 10 contractions every 10 minutes. Caldeyro-Barcia (1969) reported that intramammary pressure rose 10 mmHg at five days postpartum during oxytocin release. Drewett, Bowen-Jones, & Dogterom (1982) and McNeilly, Robinson, Houston, & Howie (1983) have shown by minute-to-minute blood sampling that oxytocin release occurs in impulses at about one-minute intervals. Similar results have been seen using diagnostic ultrasound to identify widening of the lactiferous ducts, indicating a milk ejection, both during breastfeeding and when using an electric breast pump (Ramsay et al., 2006). Thus oxytocin release is pulsatile and variable, with intermittent bursts, and such a pattern is seen not only with an infant at breast, but also when a mother uses a breast pump. Measurements by ultrasound of intervals between milk ejections averages 123 seconds between the beginning of each duct dilatation, with different mothers showing differing patterns, but individual mothers demonstrating a consistent pattern of milk ejections (Prime, Geddes, Hepworth, Trengove, & Hartmann, 2011). These pressure changes cease when suckling or pumping stimulation ends. Oxytocin also responds in the same way to prenursing stimuli and mechanical nipple stimulation by a breast pump.

The milk-ejection reflex, initiated by oxytocin release, serves to increase the intraductal mammary pressure and maintain it at sufficient levels to overcome the resistance of the breast to the outflow of milk. There is approximately 30 to 35 ml of milk ingested by the infant per milk-ejection (Hartmann, 2002). Milk ducts stay dilated approximately 1.5 to 3.5 minutes following letdown (Hartmann, 2002), making it beneficial to elicit multiple letdowns during the course of a pumping session. Ramsey and colleagues (2006) observed that the first milk ejection of the expression period released significantly more milk than subsequent milk ejections, regardless of vacuum level. The first two milk ejections produce the greatest percentage (62%) of total milk volume during breast expression with an electric breast pump (Prime et al., 2011). There is a significant decline in the rate at which milk is removed after the initial milk ejection (Ramsay, Mitoulas, Kent, Larsson, & Hartmann, 2005). Women with the highest increase in ductal diameter and with more and longer milk ejections expressed more milk. This may provide a partial explanation of why some mothers are able to express large amounts of milk in short periods of time, and others, whose anatomy may preclude to small ducts that do not dilate to a great extent and who do not experience as many let downs during pumping, may express lesser amounts of milk. The variable patterns of milk ejection that have been identified may have further implications for mothers using a breast pump such that pumping guidelines might be created that are more individualized. For example, mothers with a more continuous flow of milk whose milk ejections are large and late in the pumping session would take longer than eight minutes to express most of the milk in their breasts, while mothers with faster milk ejections that occur earlier in the pumping session might need less time to express the bulk of their available milk (Prime et al., 2011).

Chapter 5. Review of the Literature

The current breast pump market offers what can be a bewildering array of hand pumps, battery-operated pumps, and electric pumps. There are frequent changes in manufacturers, in the pumps, and in the availability of differing versions of the same pump, making breast pump selection somewhat arduous. There are few guidelines and little research in how to help mothers choose the best pump for their needs. Guidelines are often offered by pump manufacturers in terms of which of their own brand of pump to use. Typical advice is for mothers to use a hand pump if they will be pumping only occasionally, a personal-use electric pump for regular pumping, such as with employed mothers, and a hospital-grade, multi-user pump if they have a preterm or ill infant or if they are completely pump dependent. Breast pump ratings by mothers can be found on several websites[25, 26, 27] and may give the clinician some background on pump performance, problems, or effectiveness, but do not really provide an evidence-based resource for recommendations. Mothers' opinions of pumps are highly subjective. A number of studies have compared various pumps to each other. Clinicians may be helped by some of these comparisons and characteristics, but because pumps change so frequently, older studies may have looked at pumps that have had changes in their features or are no longer on the market. The varying methodologies among these studies further complicate decision-making.

- Fewtrell, Lucas, Collier, Singhal, Ahluwalia, and Lucas (2001) compared the Isis manual pump (Canon Avent) to the Ameda hospital-grade double-electric pump in mothers of preterm infants. Mothers expressed milk three to four times per day and spent less time pumping with the double electric pump than the single manual pump. The total volume of milk expressed over the study period was greater in the electric pump group than in the manual pump group. When pumping sequentially (one breast at a time), the manual pump group was found to yield significantly greater milk flow and total volume over 20 minutes than the electric pump group. The calculated volume of milk per breast per minute was slightly higher in the manual pump group, indicating greater milk flow. It is unknown if user hand fatigue would

---

25 http://www.epinions.com/kifm-Baby_Equipment/submitted_form_~ultrafinder/ultrafinder_ submitted_~%20Go%20/skp_~1/dl_~1/search_vertical_~all/search_string_~breast%20pumps

26 http://www.amazon.com/s/ref=nb_sb_noss?url=search-alias%3Dhpc&field-keywords=breast+pumps&x=0&y=0

27 http://www.breastpumpcomparisons.com/

have come in to play if the mothers had been pumping more times per day and/or over a more extended period of time. Mothers rated the manual pump higher on five consumer characteristics - ease of use, amount of suction, comfort, pleasant to use, and overall opinion. The study was funded by the manufacturer of the manual pump.

• Fewtrell, Lucas, Collier, and Lucas (2001) conducted a study that compared the manual Isis breast pump (Canon Avent) to the Mini-electric pump (Medela) in term mothers tested on a single occasion. Each mother tested both pumps once for a 20-minute test period, with 10 minutes of pumping on each breast. The volume of milk pumped was similar for both pumps. The Isis pump received better scores on three of the five consumer characteristics (comfort, pleasant to use, and overall opinion of the pump) compared with the Mini-electric pump, which scored better on ease of use and amount of suction. It is difficult to make a judgment on either of these pumps since the study protocol only had the mothers use the pump once. The study was funded by the manufacturer of the manual pump.

• Hayes et al. (2008) conducted a study to determine whether an electric breast pump or a manual pump would increase breastfeeding duration in mothers returning to work or school full time. The use of an electric breast pump did not differ statistically from the use of a manual pump in overall duration of breastfeeding. Although the same information and support was given to all mothers in the study, additional support was required in some cases for women in the manual pump group. Some crossover occurred with a number of mothers in the manual pump group also using an electric pump unbeknownst to the researchers. The authors claim that the findings suggest that the manual breast pump may work as well as the electric breast pump when breastfeeding is encouraged and supported among women returning to work or school. The findings may not warrant such a claim as mothers in the manual pump group had used an electric pump, raising questions about the conclusion.

• Meier et al. (2008) conducted a study to compare the efficiency, efficacy, comfort, and convenience of three different suction patterns used in the new Symphony breast pump (Medela) including a multi-phased pattern, compared to the single phase pattern used in the Classic breast pump (Medela) in mothers of preterm infants. Single-phase suction patterns in an electric pump use a uniform repeating cycle of suction and release. Multiphase patterns employ varying speeds and intensities of suction and release cycles that are purported to mimic the breastfeeding infant. The time to milk ejection was significantly shorter for the single versus the multiphase patterns. No other statistically significant differences were found among the suction patterns for any of the other measures of efficiency, including total pumping time, milk output at five minute intervals, percentage of total milk output at five minutes intervals, and speed of milk flow. The multiphase pump was as efficient and effective as the single-phase pump, but was deemed more comfortable to use by the mothers. The study was partially funded by the manufacturer of the two pumps.

- Hopkinson and Heird (2009) compared the prolactin response to pumping using two different electric breast pumps (Embrace by Playtex and Pump In Style by Medela). The researchers found that the prolactin response was greater with the Embrace pump, but milk extraction efficiency was greater with the Pump In Style breast pump, which extracted more milk with a higher fat content in 10 minutes of pumping. The pumps did not differ in their ability to increase milk production over time or in their ability to support long-term milk production. The authors discussed how the Embrace pump stimulated the endocrine half of the milk production system, while the Pump In Style stimulated the autocrine arm. While the mothers in the study alternately used both pumps during the study period, they were no more likely to choose one pump over the other in terms of which pump they chose to keep. The two pumps seemed comparable for long-term ability to support adequate milk production when using the pump twice per day.

- Sisk, Quandt, Parson, and Tucker (2010) looked at factors that supported or hindered initiation and maintenance of breastmilk expression after the birth of a very low birth weight infant. Mothers who relied on small electric or manual pumps to express their milk after being discharged from the hospital reported great difficulty in establishing an effective pumping schedule and an adequate milk supply. This was reported as being due to the pumps being painful, tiring to use, and ineffective at emptying the breasts. Some mothers were too weak to manually pump milk, resulting in several days with no milk expression.

- Clark and Dellaport (2011) looked at the efficacy of issuing a multi-user electric breast pump compared to a single-user electric breast pump (Medela) to mothers in the Special Supplemental Nutrition Program for Women, Infants and Children (WIC) who were separated from their infants for greater than 30 hours per week during work or school. With the single-user breast pump, less WIC formula was issued and less WIC staff time was needed to issue the breast pumps. Total formula costs for the multi-user electric pump group who chose to supplement with formula amounted to $8564.77 for the year compared to the single-user breast pump group whose formula costs amounted to $5287.16 for the year. The single-user breast pump group appeared to increase the duration of offering breastmilk to the WIC participant's infants.

- Wight, Turfler, Grassley, and Spencer (2011) evaluated the milk production of preterm mothers using a small multi-user breast pump (P.J.'s Comfort pump) with the features of the larger, more expensive multi-user breast pumps. In this study, 83% of mothers using this pump achieved > 350mL/d of expressed milk, 66% achieved > 500mL/d, and 29% pumped > 700mL/d, which are volumes compatible with the ability to supply adequate amounts of milk over the long term to premature infants (Hill, Aldag, Chatterton, & Zinaman, 2005; Meier et al., 2011). The authors state that this pump is a viable alternative to the larger, more expensive electric pumps and provides yet another option for mothers of preterm infants to acquire an efficient pump that will initiate and maintain their milk production.

Some studies have looked at various characteristics of pumps in an effort to build in evidence-based features that would result in better efficiency, improved milk output, and increased comfort. The studies below were fully or partially funded by Medela.

- Mitoulas et al. (2002b) developed a procedure to study several parameters of breast pump efficacy (time to milk ejection, amount of milk removed, and rate of milk removal) in a computerized pump programmed to operate like the Medela Classic electric breast pump. The mean volume of milk expressed was related to the degree of fullness of the breast. The authors found that the rate of milk expression changed over the course of a five-minute expression period, staying constant for the first 2.5 minutes, but decreasing by the five-minute mark. There was great variation between mothers, with some being able to pump a large amount of milk quickly and others taking much longer to pump milk.

- Kent, Ramsay, Doherty, Larsson, and Hartmann (2003) assessed the effectiveness of differing stimulation patterns provided by an electric breast pump, as well as the volume of milk removed, the changes in the lactiferous ducts in the breast, and the mothers' perceptions of the differing suction patterns. An infant stimulates the milk ejection reflex at the start of a feeding by engaging in rapid sucking, between 72 and 120 sucks per minute, before slowing to approximately 60 sucks per minute once the milk ejection reflex as been activated and milk begins to flow. The authors found that each milk ejection makes a certain amount of milk available, and the applied vacuum affects how fast this amount is removed.

• Kent et al. (2008) studied the effect of the strength of vacuum on the total milk yield and rate of milk flow from the breast. Using the two-phase cycling pattern of the Symphony double electric breast pump (Medela), mothers started pumping at 125 cycles per minute at a vacuum level that was comfortable. After the milk ejection reflex was detected, the pump pattern was changed to the expression pattern of 54–78 cycles per minute and the vacuum was adjusted to the maximum at which the mother was comfortable. Expressing milk at the mother's maximum comfort vacuum yielded more milk, resulted in faster expression of the milk, and pumped more of the available milk than when using lower vacuums. To help maximize milk yield and minimize pumping time, mothers can be advised to use their own maximum amount of comfortable vacuum as soon as the milk ejection reflex is detected. It was also shown that most of the milk is expressed following the first two milk ejections and that expression using the maximum comfortable vacuum for eight minutes may be a sufficient amount of time to pump, which is especially important for mothers who must pump milk in a short period of time, such as employed mothers with short break times. Some mothers in this study, however, were not able to remove a significant proportion of the available milk in their breasts using certain vacuum and cycling patterns. This could be a function of some mothers actually needing more vacuum than the 270 mmHg maximum that the experimental pump could generate. Milk output can be improved in such a situation with the addition of breast massage while pumping to create a more effective pressure gradient between breast and pump. Breast massage will increase the positive pressure within the breast rather than having to increase vacuum, which can be painful to the mother or damage the nipple.

• Prime et al. (2009) used an experimental system to study whether milk ejections occurred simultaneously in both breasts during double pumping with an electric breast pump. The study found that the left and right breasts responded with simultaneous milk ejection 95.5% of the time. There was no advantage shown for regulating vacuum levels separately for each breast during double expression. The percentage of available milk removed varied by almost 25% on average between the left and right breasts of a mother, despite the same amount of vacuum being applied to both breasts.

- Engstrom, Janes, Jegier, and Loera (2012) compared the effectiveness, efficiency, comfort, and convenience of new breast pump suction patterns for mothers of preterm infants. The new suction pattern was designed to mimic the rapid sucking rate and irregular sucking rhythm used by healthy term infants during breastfeeding before the onset of lactogenesis II, when only small amounts of milk are available for removal. The new suction pattern was compared to the Symphony two-phase (2.0) pattern in the Symphony double electric breast pump (Medela). The new pattern provided an intensive rapid rate stimulus and burst-pause pattern and was found to be effective in mothers in achieving significantly greater milk output over the study period compared to the two-phase pattern. Starting on day 8 of the study, the mothers using the experimental suction pattern demonstrated significantly greater cumulative milk output, and the difference continued throughout the rest of the study period. A greater percentage of mothers using the experimental pattern achieved both > 350mL/day by day 7 and > 500mL/day on day 11, 12, and 14.

- Prime, Kent, Hepworth, Trengove, and Hartmann (2011) found that the maximum flow rate of milk during pumping occurred at either the first or second milk ejection 94% of the time. Long milk expression periods (15 minutes or more) may not be necessary for most mothers. Although there was no difference between the 24-hour milk production between the left and right breasts, 46% of the mothers in the study had one breast that produced at least 25% less milk than the other breast. In the study mothers, milk flowed more quickly in the first seven minutes of expression, with 80% of the milk volume removed in the first six minutes for most mothers. The study found that there is a stronger milk flow from fuller breasts, but a larger proportion of milk remains in these breasts after pumping, reinforcing the advice that for increased pumping effectiveness, mothers should avoid long intervals between milk removal.

Chapter 6. The Pumps

There are a plethora of pumps currently on the market, each with its pros and cons. Table 6.1 provides a general summary of the differing pumps.

Table 6.1. Comparison of Pump Types

Type of Pump

TYPE OF PUMP	PROS	CONS	GOOD FOR
HAND	Light, small, portable, less expensive, do not require batteries or electricity, quiet, fewer parts to break	Empty only one breast at a time, may result in user fatigue, not for women with carpal tunnel syndrome, arthritis, or other hand or arm problems, may be less efficient and more time consuming to use, limited flange sizes	Situations where there is no electricity or access to an electric pump, useful as a backup to electric pump, useful for occasional pumping or short absences from baby, useful for limited applications like engorgement
PEDAL	Does not require electricity or batteries, can be used by mothers with hand or arm problems, less expensive than large electric pumps	Can be awkward to transport	Useful for occupations or environments where no electricity is available and mother needs to pump multiple times per day

Type of Pump	Pros	Cons	Good for
Battery	Small, portable, less expensive than electric pumps, do not require electricity, many have AC adapters to run on electricity, may be more effective when AC adapter is used	Can be noisy, some break easily, limited warranty and lifetime, may cycle slower with lower vacuum, can be expensive with frequent battery replacement, empty only one breast at a time, limited flange sizes	Useful for occasional pumping or as a backup for an electric pump
Electric	Cycling and vacuum closer to that of a nursing infant, longer warranties and lifetime, empty both breasts at the same time, faster milk expression, AC adapters and battery options, can be rented, some pumps offer multiple flange sizes, some are approved as multi-user	Expensive, heavy, can be noisy, requires source of electricity, small electric pumps may have ineffective vacuum and cycling patterns, as well as limited motor life, single user pumps should not be shared	Hospital-grade and personal-use pumps have a good history for mothers needing frequent pumping over long periods of time; small electric pumps may not be suitable for heavy duty pumping
Avent	27.0 mm 24.0 mmStandard Insert		
Hygeia	27.0 mmStandard		

Hand or Manual Pumps

The various types of hand pumps rely on differing mechanisms to generate suction.

Bicycle Horn and Rubber Bulb Breast Pumps

Rubber bulb pumps are seldom seen or used in current clinical practice. Squeezing and releasing a rubber bulb generates a vacuum in these pumps. The rubber bulb is generally attached directly to the collection reservoir, allowing for the easy backflow of milk into the rubber bulb. This poses a significant risk for bacterial contamination, as the inside of the rubber bulb cannot be sufficiently cleaned. Mothers complain that this type of pump lacks sufficient vacuum, vacuum generation is unreliable, the rubber bulb often has an unpleasant odor, and the pumped milk sometimes smells and tastes like the rubber bulb. There is little control over how much vacuum is generated and the small milk collection reservoir, which may hold as little as one-half ounce of milk, must be emptied very frequently into another container. The flange comes in only one size, which means that it may not provide a good fit for some mothers. Because vacuum is generated by squeezing and releasing the rubber bulb, mothers may find this tiring. Women with carpal tunnel syndrome, arthritis, or any other problem with their hands, wrists, or arms may find this pump both difficult and painful to use. Mothers might find this pump useful to relieve engorgement if there is no other pump available, but hand expression in that situation would offer a much better option. A major concern with this type of pump is its unproven ability to sustain high milk production when used over a longer period of time. Because there are so many other pumps that have features better suited to long-term pumping, the bicycle horn pump would likely be a poor choice for most mothers and situations. This type of pump, such as the Nuby On-the-Go, can easily be found on the Internet. Reviews are sparse and not very good at this time. Some manufacturers separate the bulb from the collection container by modifying the angle at which it is attached to the pump or by adding a length of tubing. These modifications are thought to reduce the high potential for bacterial contamination of the bulb caused by the easy backflow of milk. Backflow risk is reduced when the bulb is separated from the collection container.

Squeeze-Handle Models

Squeeze-handle models involve squeezing and releasing a handle that creates suction in the pump, such as the Harmony (Medela), the Ameda One Hand, Simplisse manual, Philips Avent Isis manual, Lansinoh manual,

Playtex manual, and the Evenflo Simply Go. The Hygeia manual breast pump uses a plunger within a cylinder that is pushed and pulled to generate vacuum. These types of pumps are typically used for occasional pumping, and can be used when no electricity is available or for ease when traveling. These pumps are easily cleaned, but their operation may present difficulties for women with hand or arm problems, such as arthritis or carpal tunnel syndrome. The hand and wrist can tire easily with repeated use. Mothers have mixed reviews about many of these pumps, with a number of complaints that some of the pumps break easily and some do not generate enough vacuum, while other reviewers love some of these pumps for occasional pumping or mention certain features of a particular pump that make pumping easier or more efficient. The vacuum on some of the pumps can be unreliable, while other hand pumps generate dependable vacuum throughout their use and have safeguards that prevent too much vacuum from being generated. Cycling of the vacuum depends on how fast the mother squeezes the handle and how long she holds it. Some mothers use an electric pump while at work and one of the hand pumps when traveling or out of the house. Some mothers who work in conditions where there is not consistent access to electrical outlets (mothers in the military, police officers, transportation workers, construction and other outdoor occupations) use two hand pumps (or battery pumps) simultaneously to decrease pumping time and improve milk output.

Battery-Operated Pumps

Battery-operated pumps use a small motor, with usually either size AA 1.5-volt batteries or size C batteries to generate the power, such as the Mini Electric (Medela). These pumps are designed for short term, limited use. Most have a vacuum adjustment mechanism, so mothers can adjust the vacuum to their comfort level. Vacuum in some pumps can take a longer time to reach maximum level and is regulated by how frequently the vacuum is interrupted. Some of the pumps have automatic cycling. All take varying periods of time for the recovery of suction following each release. This limits the number of suction/release cycles per minute and may require relatively long periods of vacuum application to the nipple. To compensate for this, some mothers leave the suction on for much longer than the pump instructions recommend. One manufacturer recommends that the pump be used no more than twice per day.

Most battery-operated pumps have AC adapters available to plug into an electrical outlet, which decreases battery use. A major complaint about these pumps is their short battery life, with mothers having to constantly purchase more batteries. This affects pumping efficiency because fewer cycles are generated as the batteries wear down. Batteries may have to be replaced as frequently as every second or third use. Rechargeable batteries are an option, but they usually require charging each night and may not produce as many cycles per minute as alkaline batteries. AC adapters usually allow the maximum number of cycles per minute that the motor can produce, but require access to an electrical outlet, negating some of the advantages of portability. Maximum suction after each vacuum release can in some pumps continue decreasing in amount throughout the pumping session. Cycling is preset and can be adjusted in some pumps.

Battery pumps require only one hand to operate and are lightweight. Some mothers use two battery-operated pumps simultaneously, one on each breast, to decrease pumping time when they are on a tight schedule. Mothers who plan to pump for several months while at work might do better to consider using a personal-use larger electric pump or a long-term rental electric pump, because battery replacement can be very expensive–– as can artificial formula if it must be used to substitute for breastmilk. Some of the pumps operate with a quiet hum, while others are very noisy. Many mothers have unrealistic expectations regarding the efficiency and longevity of these pumps. The small motors will not operate in the same manner and length of time that is seen in the larger personal-use electric pumps. Clinicians may need to make sure mothers know that even though many of these pumps are advertised as electric pumps, they are not equivalent to the larger personal-use or hospital-grade multi-user pumps.

Electric Pumps

Electric breast pumps fall into one of three categories:

- Small semiautomatic pumps, such as the Nurture III (Bailey Medical).

- Personal-use pumps (light-weight portable pumps often used by employed mothers), such as the Pump In Style (Medela), Ameda Purely Yours, Enjoye (Hygeia), and Simplisse double electric. Some other small electric pumps are also available, but are not designed for heavy use over long periods of time, such as the Freestyle and Swing (Medela), Simply Go single and duo (Evenflo), Lansinoh double electric, Playtex Petite double electric breast pump, miPump (The First Years), and the Avent twin and single electronic pump (Philips Avent).

- Hospital-grade, multi-user pumps, such as the Symphony and Lactina (Medela), Platinum and Elite (Ameda), EnDeare (Hygeia), and P.J.'s Comfort (Limerick).

The Nurture III semiautomatic pump uses manual cycling that requires the mother to cycle suction by covering and uncovering a vent in one of the collection bottles, a process that creates a pumping rhythm that is controlled by the mother rather than preset in the pump. Semiautomatic pumps maintain a constant negative pressure. Some mothers learn to roll their finger three-fourths of the way off the hole rather than lift the finger completely, to generate vacuum faster for the subsequent cycle by preventing complete interruption of vacuum. However, too much negative pressure or negative pressure applied for too long a period increases the risk of damage to the nipple and underlying vascular structures. The initiation of suction places the greatest pressure on the nipple; thus, it is most desirable that a pump generate suction quickly. The Nurture III reaches 220 mmHg in two to three seconds, allowing 20-30+ cycles per minute. This is about half of what large multi-user pumps are capable of generating. This pump uses alternating vacuum, pumping one breast, and then the other.

Most automatic electric pumps are designed to cycle vacuum rather than to maintain it without interruption. Because Egnell (1956) observed nipple damage when cycles were two seconds long (30 per minute), manufacturers increased the number of cycles generated per minute to reduce the likelihood of pain or damage to the nipples. Vacuum setting parameters on these large pumps also attempt to stay within the range of the vacuum an infant generates, without exceeding what would normally be seen in an infant at the breast. Mean sucking pressures of most full-term infants range from 50 to 155 mmHg, with a maximum of approximately 220 mmHg (Caldeyro-Barcia, 1969; Mizuno & Ueda, 2006). Mothers have a wide range of tolerability for various vacuum settings. Kent et al. (2008) found that half of the mothers in their study on vacuum and milk expression were comfortable using a vacuum stronger than 200 mmHg, but one mother could not use a vacuum higher than 98 mmHg. In pumps that have a preset pulsed suction (automatic pumps), there is typically a 60/40 ratio. Negative pressure is applied for 60 percent of the cycle; 40 percent of the cycle is the resting phase. The Medela Symphony operates with a "stimulation" phase at the start of the pumping session at 120 cycles per minute, with variable adjustable vacuum of 50 to 200 mmHg. Then changes to the "expression" phase to cycle between 54 to 78 cycles per minute, with vacuum from 50 to 250 mmHg. The number of cycles per minute varies in this pump according to the set vacuum, with higher vacuum levels resulting in lower cycles per minute. At a minimum vacuum of 50 mmHg, the Symphony applies 78 cycles per minute, and at the maximum vacuum of 250 mmHg, 54 cycles per minute are applied. The maximum pressure that these pumps will generate at their normal (high) setting is approximately 220 to 250 mmHg. The Symphony pump also has what is called the Preemie Card, which contains three patterns of expressing and is used by mothers of preterm infants (Pattern 1 is 70-120 mmHg at 120 cycles per minute to stimulate milk ejection, Pattern 2 is 70-200 mmHg at 90 cycles per minute, and Pattern 3 is 100-200 mmHg at 34-54 cycles per minute). These cycles rotate with pauses. The Simplisse electric pump generates a continuous "latch" vacuum of about 30 mmHg. The vacuum range on the Simplisse Double Electric pump is from 75 to 175 mmHg and cycles from 40 to 80 cycles per minute. The latch pressure is approximately 30 mmHg and the compression pressure is approximately 100 mmHg. Rather than the vacuum and release pattern found in other electric pumps, the Simplisse pump uses compression to express breast milk. The breast cup is flat and pliable. The outer breast cup of the two-part breast cup gently compresses against the areola, while the inner breast cup produces a fluttering motion (or squeeze). The suction curve is symmetrical.

Negative pressure is a function of the volume of air in the accessory kit. It increases as the collection bottle fills with milk. The pressure generated varies with different sized bottles (collecting containers). When double-pump setups are used (with two collecting containers being filled simultaneously), the potential for very low negative pressure exists when the containers are empty; negative pressure increases as the bottles fill. Most accessory kits compensate for this by separating the collection containers from the power source, so the amount of air in the system remains constant, regardless of the amount of fluid in the collection container. Thus vacuum pressures are not dependent on air in the system and will not vacillate excessively during a pumping session. If a mother is using an accessory kit or pump without a similar feature, she can compensate by using a smaller collection bottle (Vol-u-feeders fit on some pumps), turning down the vacuum as the bottle fills, emptying the bottle more frequently, or cycling the suction more frequently on the hand, battery-operated, or semiautomatic pumps. The Simplisse pump has soft flanges that pulsate at speeds set by the mother. It does not use alternating vacuum pulses, but has inner flange liners that rhythmically compress the breast.

Chapter 7. Simultaneous or Sequential Pumping

All of the electric pumps and some of the battery-operated pumps have collection kits that allow the mother to pump both breasts at the same time. A number of studies have been conducted on the effects of simultaneous pumping compared with sequential pumping.

- Neifert and Seacat (1985) described the experiences of 10 mothers who were two to seven months postpartum. The women alternated between sequentially pumping each breast for 20 minutes, and then pumping both breasts simultaneously for 10 minutes. Milk volume was similar between both techniques, but was obtained in one-half the time with lower pump suction (320 mmHg versus 260 mmHg) when pumping was simultaneous. There was a significantly higher prolactin rise with double pumping compared with pumping one breast at a time.

- Auerbach (1990) studied 25 mothers whose infants were between five and 35 weeks of age regarding the milk yield between single and double pumping. Also studied was whether it takes longer to pump with a single setup compared to a double setup, and whether the milk fat varies between the two methods of pumping. The highest milk yields with single pumping was seen over a pumping period of 10 to 15 minutes. With double pumping, maximum milk volumes were seen in seven to 12 minutes. The highest overall volume of milk that was pumped occurred with double pumping. When asked, the mothers preferred double pumping three to one.

- Groh-Wargo et al. (1995) studied 32 preterm mothers, half of whom pumped each breast in sequence; the other half pumped both breasts simultaneously. Daily frequency of pumping in both groups ranged from three to nearly five times. The single pumping group averaged 24 minutes for each pumping session; the bilateral pumping group expressed milk for an average of 16 minutes per session. A number of factors combined to result in optimum milk expression: vacuum generated by the pump, cycling patterns of the vacuum, compressive forces from the pump flange, compressive forces external to the pump, oxytocin pulses, sequential or simultaneous pumping, number of times per day and per week of pumping sessions, time postpartum when pumping was initiated, type of flange, proper fit of the flange, comfort, etc.

- Hill, Aldag, & Chatterton (1996) conducted a small study of mothers who pumped five to seven times per day, either sequentially or simultaneously with a Lactina electric breast pump (Medela). The sequential group's milk yield was higher on day 21 of the study, as was the prolactin level, while the simultaneous group's prolactin response and milk yield was higher on day 42 and continued to increase. The simultaneous system was favored by mothers, as it decreased the time spent pumping.

- Hill, Aldag, & Chatterton (1999) studied 39 mothers of preterm infants to compare milk production from either sequential pumping or simultaneous pumping with a Lactina electric breast pump (Medela). Milk weight was higher in the simultaneous group during each week of the study, but not statistically significant. Higher milk yields can serve as an incentive to continue pumping over a longer period of time, which is especially important for pump-dependent mothers of preterm or ill infants or infants who cannot feed at the breast. Even though the two methods did not produce significantly different milk yields, the mothers using sequential pumping required 20 minutes per pumping session to express their milk, while mothers in the simultaneous group required a minimum of 10 minutes. The difference in time commitment can have a significant influence on the willingness of mothers to continue pumping over prolonged periods of time. It is interesting that in spite of the advantages of simultaneous pumping, some mothers in this study preferred sequential pumping because it left them with a free hand to engage in other activities while pumping.

- Jones, Dimmock, & Spencer (2001) looked at preterm mothers to compare sequential (19 mothers) with simultaneous breast pumping (17 mothers) on milk volume and energy yield. Also compared was the effect of breast massage on milk volume and energy yield. Mothers used an Ameda Elite electric breast pump. Mothers pumped a mean frequency of five times per day. Simultaneous pumping with or without massage was more effective than single pumping in producing an increased volume of milk and a higher fat content. From a single pumping session:

  ▷ Sequential, non-massage = 46 to 56 mL

  ▷ Sequential, massage = 73 to 85 mL

▷ Simultaneous, non-massage = 79 to 97 mL

▷ Simultaneous, massage = 110 to 140 mL

Simultaneous pumping in this study was able to compensate for the typical low-milk production in preterm mothers.

Chapter 8. Flanges

Most pumps or pump collection kits have hard plastic shields called flanges into which the nipple and areola are drawn during pumping. There are a variety of flanges, with some pumps having softer plastic or silicone flanges, soft inner liners, soft inserts, hard inserts, projections on the flange that purport to compress the breast when vacuum is applied, or other types of inserts that change the diameter of the nipple opening.

Johnson (1983) measured a number of aspects of flanges, including the diameter of the outer opening (flare), the diameter of the inner opening, the depth of the flare, and the length of the shank. She also measured the amount of negative pressure at the inner opening of the flange and found that the smaller the nipple cup the greater the pressure that was exerted on the tip of the nipple. Johnson speculated that the larger and deeper flanges could provide greater stimulation of the areolar region of the breast. Zinaman (1988) repeated the same measurements on 11 manual pumps, four battery pumps, and seven electric pumps. The diameter of the flange ranged from 60 to 69 mm, depth ranged from 25 to 30 mm, and the inner opening was between 21 and 26 mm for the manual pumps. A woman with a large or wide nipple could have difficulty with a flange that has a small opening or a narrow slope, as many of these older pumps demonstrated.

Because one size of flange is not appropriate for all breasts, some manufacturers provide a choice of different sized flanges (Table 8.1), silicone flange liners, or small plastic inserts that are placed at the level of the inner opening to change the diameter of the shank and inner opening for a better fit. Silicone or soft plastic flange liners are marketed by pump manufacturers to cushion the pumping forces and are purported to "massage" the breast or mimic external compressive forces. Inserts placed in some flanges are designed to narrow the inner opening of the flange to provide a better fit between pump and breast.

Table 8.1. Breast Pump Flange Sizes

	Extra small insert	21.0 mm
	Small insert	22.5 mm
	Standard	25.0 mm
	Medium	28.5 mm
	Large	30.5 mm
	XL	32.5 mm
	XXL	36.0 mm
	Standard Insert	27.0 mm
		24.0 mm
	Standard	27.0 mm
	Small	21.0 mm
	Standard	24.0 mm
	Large	27.0 mm
	XL	30.0 mm
	XXL	36.0 mm
	Blown glass	40.0 mm
	Original	23-29 mm
	Large	29-35 mm
	XL	35 mm+

When vacuum is applied, the nipple and part of the areola elongate and are drawn past the inner opening and down into the shank or nipple tunnel (Biancuzzo, 1999). In general, pumping is more likely to be effective when the flange accommodates the anatomic configuration of the particular breast. However, mothers have various sized nipples. Ziemer and Pigeon (1993), Stark (1994), and Wilson-Clay and Hoover (2005) measured nipple diameters, finding a wide range, from <12 mm at base to >23 mm at base. Wilson-Clay and Hoover (2005) also observed that nipples swell during pumping. Using a circle template, the authors took pre- and post-pumping measurements of the nipple, showing that it can increase in size by as much as 3 to 4 mm during a pumping session. As a comparison, the pre-pumping nipple was about the size of a US nickel, while after pumping the nipple was about the size of a U.S. quarter. This can pose a problem for a mother with large nipples, as she may find that a standard size flange is too small to accommodate both the larger nipple and the subsequent swelling during pumping. Meier, Motyhowski, & Zuleger (2004) studied a sample of mothers expressing milk for their preterm infants. The authors noted that about half of the mothers required a 27–30 mm flange, rather than the standard 23–24 mm flange that comes with most electric pumping collection kits. As lactation progressed in these mothers, 77% of the mothers found they needed a larger flange. Damage has been observed by clinicians on the areola, sometimes presenting as suction rings or cracks at the junction of the nipple and areola, from flanges that are too small. Nipples can also become abraded from rubbing against the pump flange. Such a misfit between flange and breast can endanger milk production if the teat is strangulated to the point where little to no milk can be expressed. Wilson-Clay and Hoover (2005) speculate that if a mother has a nipple size of approximately 20.5 mm (or the size of a US nickel) or larger, she may benefit from using a larger than standard size pump flange. There are no clinical algorithms for flange selection based on nipple size that allow clinicians to advise mothers on which size flange to use. If the nipple is 20 mm in diameter or larger, the mother may be advised to use one size larger than the standard flange. Some health professionals who have access to autoclaving or similar sterilizing facilities offer mothers the opportunity to try several different brands of breast pumps and flange sizes in order to determine an optimal fit before a pump is purchased or rented. Some mothers who have difficulty with any of the numerous sized flanges provided by the pump manufacturers find they can achieve a good fit between their nipples that change size during the pumping session when they use an angled flange called the Pumpin Pal Super Shield (Figure 8.1). This angled flange comes in three sizes and fits into the pump's own flange as an insert. The set of three flanges allows mothers to use whatever size works best. Some mothers rotate these flanges during the day or over time. The flange allows the mother to sit upright or slightly reclined while pumping and often provides a good fit when no other flanges are working well for the mother.

Figure.8.1. Pumpin Pal Angled Flange

A properly fitted flange has enough space between the nipple and the inner walls so the nipple moves freely back and forth during pumping, but not so much space that too much of the areola is also drawn down into the shank of the flange. If the flange is too tight, it may impede adequate drainage of the breast. Residual milk that is not removed can gradually contribute to downregulation of the milk supply, provide the potential for plugged milk ducts, increase the formation of focal points of engorgement, and ultimately contribute to mastitis in some mothers.

Jones et al. (2001) found that almost one-third of the 36 women in their study of preterm pumping mothers experienced disparity in the fit between their nipple and the size of the pump flange's nipple tunnel. Pump flanges can also be too large, which can contribute to nipple pain and damage to the areola. Some mothers may find they need a different size shield for each breast, and/or that as lactation progresses, they actually need a smaller size flange (Jones & Hilton, 2009). It can take some experimentation to find the correctly fitting flange. Mothers or clinicians can measure the nipple size at the base of the nipple. Fitting guidelines should take the following into account.

A mother may need a larger flange if:

- The nipple rubs against the side of the nipple tunnel or sticks to the side. This can be painful and abrade the nipple over time. Pain can interfere with milk ejection and contribute to diminished amounts of milk being pumped.

- The nipple does not move freely in the tunnel after about five minutes of pumping. This indicates the nipple has swelled and would benefit from a larger flange. Milk ducts are very superficial and continued compression of the nipple may impede milk flow.

- The entire nipple does not fit into the nipple tunnel. This can lead to pain and damage to the nipple.

- The nipple does not move back and forth in a smooth rhythmical motion. This indicates it is sticking to the side of the nipple tunnel or the flange would benefit from lubrication with a little olive oil.

- The mother experiences nipple pain while pumping. This can indicate a poorly fitting flange or vacuum that is too high.

- The tip of the nipple becomes sore or blistered. The flange should be changed to a larger one and the amount of vacuum should be reduced if it is too high.

- There are areas of the breast that are not well drained after pumping. This can indicate compression of some of the milk ducts and a larger flange can be tried.

- A ring of sloughed skin or specks of skin are seen on the inside of the shield after pumping. This usually happens if the nipple is rubbing against the side of the nipple tunnel, rather than pulsating back and forth.

- The base of the nipple is blanching (turning white) while pumping. The nipple is strangulating in a nipple tunnel that is too small.

- There is minimal or no areolar tissue being pulled into the tunnel of the flange. The flange may be too small and needs to be re-sized.

The mother may need a smaller flange if:

- The flange does not stay in complete contact with the skin or there are gaps that would compromise suction. The flange must be in complete contact with the breast in order to create vacuum.

If the mother is pumping five to eight times per day, she may find that applying nipple cream or olive oil to the nipple and areola prior to pumping makes for a better seal and prevents abrasion of the nipple.

Kent, Geddes, Hepworth, & Hartmann (2011) studied the effect of using a warmed flange on the efficiency, effectiveness, and comfort of expressing milk with an electric breast pump. The study looked specifically at the effect of warming the areola and nipple during pumping on the time taken to milk ejection, determined if there was an interaction between warmth and strength of vacuum, determined the effect of changing temperature on milk duct diameter, and assessed mothers' perceptions of using a warmed pump flange. The results indicated that a warmed flange had no effect on the time to stimulate the first milk ejection or on the number of milk ejections. When pumping with the maximum comfortable vacuum, the warm flange compared with an ambient temperature flange resulted in a shorter time to remove 80% of the total milk yield. Using the warmed flange also resulted in a higher peak milk flow rate, a larger percentage of available milk removed at two, five, and 10 minutes after milk ejection, and positive comfort comments from the mothers. Warming the flange resulted in some significant indicators of increased milk removal, possibly related to enhanced dilatation of the milk ducts within the nipple and areola.

Chapter 9.
Parameters for Choosing a Breast Pump

Many mothers choose a breast pump based on price, while others may receive a pump as a baby shower gift. Some mothers may have little choice in terms of which breast pump is available to them (for example, pumps given or loaned through a WIC office or determined by an insurance company). Clinicians may help mothers determine the best pump for their situation using the following guide:

1. Determine the mother's situation for needing a breast pump. If a mothers wishes to pump milk no more than once or twice each day or periodically during the week, if she wishes to have a light weight portable pump when out of the house for short periods of time, or if she is feeding her infant at the breast for all or almost all of the feedings and wishes to store milk for when she goes out, then a hand pump or small electric pump may be a reasonable choice for her. The mother can be referred to one of the websites where mothers themselves review pumps. Some of these small electric pumps have a very limited life and have a history of breaking or not working well for very long. If the mother will be returning to work or school or if her infant has limited skills for feeding directly at the breast, she may wish to obtain a personal use electric pump that is better suited for heavier use. If a mother has a preterm or ill infant, if the infant cannot feed directly from the breast at all due to oral anomalies, neurological issues, etc., or if the mother is completely pump dependent, then a hospital-grade, multi-user breast pump would be her best option.

2. Look at the length of the pump's warranty. A warranty of 60 or 90 days may indicate that the manufacturer does not expect the pump to last for an extended length of time. The warranty starts at the time of purchase. If a mother bought or was given a pump during her pregnancy, the warranty may expire by the time the baby is born or soon thereafter.

3. To choose a particular pump within the above three categories, clinicians need to look at:

a. The vacuum generated by the pump. How high can the vacuum go and is there a possibility of exceeding what an infant would generate? Can the mother control the amount of vacuum the pump generates? Does the pump generate enough vacuum to be effective? Too little vacuum for some mothers will not allow adequate milk removal.

b. What is the cycling pattern(s) of the pump? How many cycles per minute can the pump generate? The pump should generate approximately 40 to 60 cycles at least. Too few cycles may apply vacuum to the nipple for exceptionally long periods of time, raising the risk of tissue damage. This cycling pattern may also not be very effective at draining the breast. Is the cycling adjustable by the mother?

c. Is the pump an open or closed system? An open system increases the chances of pump and milk contamination.

d. How effective is the pump? Hand pumps and small electric pumps can take a relatively long time to remove milk, sometimes 50% to 100% more time than a large electric pump. This exposes the nipple and areola to more vacuum and may not effectively drain most of the available milk. It may also discourage some mothers from continuing to pump their milk.

e. Is the pump easy to clean? Are there particular cleaning issues with any of the parts, such as tubing that has a high rate of condensation, or is there a possibility of drawing milk into the interior of the pump or into the motor itself? Clinicians will want to help mothers find a pump that has a low probability of this happening. If the mother is using a pump that other mothers use, such as in a hospital NICU, is there monitoring of the pump and periodic cleaning or bacteriologic oversight? Are mothers given clear instructions for cleaning their collection kit if using a large electric pump?

f. Are there options for using different size flanges to obtain the best fit between flange and breast? Clinicians can measure the mother's nipple to suggest an initial size or have the mother measure to assure that the flange will properly fit the breast.

g. Can the pump express both breasts at the same time or only one breast at a time? Some pumps possess both options. Simultaneous pumping reduces pumping time and is a good option for employed mothers with limited time for each pumping session. It is also a good option for pump-dependent mothers of ill or preterm infants.

h. Is the pump easy to obtain? Where will the mother get the pump? How long will it take to obtain it? Once the pump package is opened, it may not be returnable if it proves a poor match for the mother. Some lactation consultants have the facilities to allow mothers to trial different pumps to see which works best for them.

i. Is the pump affordable or must the mother settle for a less expensive, possibly inferior pump to her needs? Is there any program or financial help available for purchasing or renting the pump? Will the mother's insurance carrier cover the cost of a rental pump if the infant is hospitalized? Does the insurance carrier provide or cover any other pumps? Does the mother's employer provide a multi-user pump for breastfeeding employees?

j. What does the warranty cover if the mother is purchasing a pump? What invalidates the warranty? How long is the warranty? How difficult is it to obtain replacement parts? How long does it take to receive parts or a new pump?

k. Is the mother considering or using a used pump? Only FDA cleared multi-user electric breast pumps should be used by more than one mother. A previously used breast pump increases the risk of pump contamination with bacteria, viruses, and mold. Used pumps may have a motor that is no longer working at its peak performance and can jeopardize the mother's milk production. Motors in small electric and personal-use pumps have a lifetime of pumping for one infant. Mothers who purchase used pumps online should be cautioned that the words "lightly used," "used only a few times," "like new," or "gently used," can be deceptive and leaves the buyer not really knowing how heavily the pump has been used. Some of the pumps may have defects. Once purchased, most of the used pumps cannot be returned and the mother may then find herself purchasing another pump. Clinicians should discourage mothers from using borrowed, loaned, or any form of used pump.

Chapter 10.
Compliance with the International Code of Marketing of Breastmilk Substitutes

The International Code of Marketing of Breastmilk Substitutes[28] (the Code) is a set of recommendations from UNICEF and the World Health Organization (WHO) in the form of voluntary guidelines that aim to regulate the marketing of breast-milk substitutes, feeding bottles, and artificial nipples. The Code was formulated in response to the realization that poor infant feeding practices were negatively affecting the growth, health, and development of children.

The marketing of infant formula, feeding bottles, and artificial nipples that idealize their use can negatively impact breastfeeding. The Code does not restrict the manufacturing or use of these products, just how they are marketed.

While breast pumps are not within the scope of the Code, some pump companies make and/or distribute artificial nipples and infant feeding bottles, which are products covered within the scope of the code. Some breast pump manufacturers in the United States who are meeting their obligations under the Code include Ameda, Hygeia, Limerick, and Bailey Medical. Some breast pump manufacturers who are not meeting their obligations under the Code include Medela, Playtex, Lansinoh, Simplisse, The First Years, and Philips Avent. This status can change frequently as companies change their marketing strategy, purchase or sell subsidiaries, or acquire or divest themselves of infant feeding products covered under the Code. Clinicians can contact the author for a listing of breast pump companies meeting their obligations under the Code.

---

28   http://www.infactcanada.ca/int_code_toc.htm

Part 3.
Pumping Protocols and Problems

Chapter 11. Pumping Protocols

While it is important to choose the best pump to fit the mother's particular needs and situation, it is also important that the pumping protocol the mother uses is one that maximizes milk yield and minimizes potential problems. Geraghty, Davidson, Tabangin, & Morrow (2011) reported that 63% of the mothers in their study on the characteristics of mothers who expressed breastmilk early in the postpartum period had begun milk expression by the end of four weeks. Thus, it is important that mothers receive adequate information and instructions on milk expression either during the prenatal period or early in the postpartum period. Mothers who pump milk once or twice per day may find they express more milk in the morning and may want to pump after or between two of the morning feedings. Employed mothers who are pumping at work or mothers of preterm infants or ill infants will need a more structured pumping plan. Mothers will want to know how to use their chosen pump, how to maximize milk yield and minimize pumping times, and how to solve pumping problems.

Morse and Bottorff (1988) studied the emotional experiences of 61 breastfeeding mothers related to breastmilk expression. Many mothers thought expressing milk was a simple matter and were surprised that their ability to express milk was not automatic. Mothers frequently found that verbal and written instructions were unclear and confusing. Many mothers learned to express milk by trial and error. Mothers in this study found and related that generalized instructions did not necessarily work for all mothers and what worked for one mother may not work for another mother. Some mothers were embarrassed and/or frustrated when they could obtain only small amounts of milk. In the study, success with breastmilk expression increased a mother's self-confidence for women who perceived expression to be an important aspect of breastfeeding. But mothers who were unable to express milk displayed heightened feelings of inadequacy. The authors of the study recommend that when teaching mothers how to express their milk, clinicians should provide not only explicit how-to's, but also encourage private exploratory practice such that each mother finds what works best for her.

Many mothers receive and must rely on only the instructions that come with the pump. They use this as a guide in learning milk expression and handling. These instructions vary widely in their recommendations on pumping techniques, and even on the cleaning of the pump. Further confusion is possible if a mother uses more than one type of pump or pumps from different manufacturers. More problems can occur if she fails to read all of the instructions carefully or if the instructions from one manufacturer conflict with those from another. Clinicians should realize that the best breast pump will do little for a mother whose emotional needs are not met and who lacks the guidelines necessary to use the equipment properly for optimal results.

Sisk et al. (2010) conducted a qualitative study to discover the factors that supported or hindered the initiation and maintenance of breastmilk expression in mothers of preterm infants. Barriers and potential interventions for each are provided below.

- PHYSICAL AND MENTAL CHALLENGES. Many mothers experienced a pregnancy-related medical complication. Half of the mothers were treated with magnesium sulfate, and many were delivered by cesarean section. Mothers who received magnesium sulfate reported side effects from the medication that made it difficult for them to understand the pumping instructions or to pump because they felt ill. Mothers who had a cesarean section complained that pain and fatigue interfered with their ability to pump during the first few days or to remember pumping instructions. Some mothers received conflicting pumping instructions. Mothers were anxious and stressed over the preterm delivery.

  Intervention: Interventions for these issues can include helping mothers better understand and remember pumping instructions. Verbal instructions are easily forgotten, so a pumping plan should be provided in written form for both the hospital stay and once discharged. Many young mothers are comfortable using electronic technology and may remember and respond better to pumping instructions that are provided on a DVD, on a hand-held or mobile device, or even on the Internet on a site such as You Tube. These options allow a mother to review and watch pumping guidelines whenever she needs to. Continued support for pumping after hospital discharge is very important. Hospital-based support groups, Internet support groups, peer counselors, lactation consultants, periodic telephone calls, web cams in the hospital NICU, and review of pumping logs are all helpful possibilities. Pumping logs are important to assure that timely interventions are available if milk yields fall or do not increase to an adequate volume. During the hospital stay, staff nurses or the lactation consultant should make sure that mothers (especially cesarean mothers) are reminded to hand express colostrum and pump on a regular basis and that they are following the pumping plan.

- **Privacy.** Mothers described that the lack of privacy in the hospital made it difficult to pump on a regular basis. Morrison, Ludington-Hoe, & Anderson (2006) studied the number and types of interruptions seen with breastfeeding mothers in the hospital during a 12 hour span of time. Each mother-infant dyad in their study experienced an average of 54 interruptions during the 12-hour observation period or a mean of 4.5 interruptions per hour. A volume of interruptions such as this interferes with a mother's ability to learn to pump, use the pump, and pump on a frequent basis. It is difficult for mothers to tell visitors to leave, and they are embarrassed to pump in front of them. Hospital staff were described as unwilling or unable to provide the amount of privacy that mothers felt they needed in order to pump as frequently as required.

  Intervention: A number of interventions by clinicians may help improve mothers' access to privacy during their hospital stay. Some hospitals have changed their visiting hours to allow mothers to obtain more rest, breastfeed more often, or pump more frequently without concern about a constant stream of visitors. The visiting hours are restricted to one hour in the late afternoon and one hour in the evening (except for the father of the baby or siblings). Some units put a sign on the door requesting privacy when a mother needs to pump. Maternity units have clustered interruptions (such as birth certificate forms, blood work, infant hearing exams, dietary, housekeeping, etc.) into a specific block of time when mothers know there will be interruptions. Other units have a rest period during the afternoon when no interruptions are permitted except for medical necessity. Mothers will have difficulty pumping if they never know who will be walking in on them. Clinicians may need to specifically remind mothers to pump, and then arrange the environment so they can do so.

- **Acquiring a suitable breast pump.** It is important that the transition from pumping in the hospital to pumping at home go smoothly. Mothers of preterm or ill infants or infants who cannot feed directly from the breast should make arrangements for a hospital-grade multi-user pump to be available when they arrive home from the hospital. Mothers in the Sisk et al. (2010) study who relied on small electric or manual pumps had great difficulty in establishing and maintaining an adequate milk supply because the pumps were said to be painful, tiring to use, and ineffective at emptying the breast.

  Intervention: Clinicians can help assure that mothers leave the hospital with a suitable pump or that arrangements have been made for such a pump to either be picked up or delivered to the mother. Most maternity units keep a list of pump rental depots, DME vendors, or have their own pump rental/loan facilities, so there is no interruption in the initiation of lactation under less than optimal circumstances.

- **GETTING PUMPED MILK TO THE HOSPITAL.** If the infant remains hospitalized after the mother is discharged, getting the pumped milk to the hospital can be problematic for some mothers. The time taken to drive to the hospital, or worse yet depend on public transportation to bring milk to the hospital proves disruptive to pumping schedules and milk production. Mothers have been inventive in finding ways to transport their pumped milk to the hospital, especially if they live a distance away and visiting is logistically difficult. Some mothers send in their milk with hospital employees or with friends, neighbors, or family that work close to the hospital. Rush Medical Center in Chicago, IL provides taxi service for mothers of hospitalized infants to facilitate visiting and milk transport, as well as attendance at a weekly lunch and learn session with lactation department staff (Meier, Engstrom, Mingolelli, Miracle, & Keisling, 2004).

  Intervention: Assure that mothers have a mechanism to transport their milk to the hospital. Check if the hospital has a van or courier service that could be used to transport expressed breastmilk. Some mothers send in their milk with hospital employees or with friends, neighbors, or family that work close to the hospital. Rush Medical Center in Chicago, IL, provides taxi service for mothers of hospitalized infants to facilitate visiting and milk transport, as well as attendance at a weekly lunch and learn session with lactation department staff (Meier, Engstrom, Mingolelli, Miracle, & Keisling, 2004).

- **MANAGING TIME.** The time it takes each day to pump can be burdensome on mothers, especially if they are caring for other children or must return to work. Pumping can conflict with eating, sleeping, taking care of oneself and the family, meeting with the infant's medical team if the infant is still hospitalized, and just leaving the house for errands or other commitments. Rather than establishing a rigid pumping schedule of every so many hours, some mothers find it easier to pump the recommended minimum of eight times each 24 hours if completely pump dependent by aiming to pump when they have a window of 10 minutes or so. Infants feeding directly from the breast feed erratically, sometimes going for longer periods of time and sometimes clustering or bunching their feedings.

Intervention: Clinicians can help mothers assemble a pumping plan for what will work best in each individual situation. Explore what forms of help are available to the mother from family, friends, neighbors, and faith and community based organizations. Rather than establishing a rigid pumping schedule of every so many hours, some mothers find it easier to pump the recommended minimum of eight times each 24 hours if completely pump dependent by aiming to pump when they have a window of 10 minutes or so. Infants feeding directly from the breast feed erratically, sometimes going for longer periods of time and sometimes clustering or bunching their feedings.

- PUMPING ATTITUDE. Some mothers found pumping to be boring and were better able to maintain frequent pumping if they did something else while pumping, such as watching television, reading, or playing video games. Mothers who double pump can free both hands by wearing a pumping bra with holes cut out for securing the pump flange to the breast. Some collection kits have straps to secure the flange to the bra. This may allow mothers to operate electronic devices, read to siblings, and take care of some household responsibilities, such as paying bills and making phone calls. Other mothers find pumping sessions to be an opportunity for solace within a hectic schedule. Mothers often plan their day around their pumping schedule.

Intervention: Clinicians may need to help mothers find the time to pump and offer suggestions found in the clinical scenarios in Chapter 13.

Chapter 12.
Facilitating More Effective Pumping

The environment surrounding pumping has been shown to have an effect on the success of pumping and a positive outcome on direct feeding of preterm infants at the breast. Furman, Minich, & Hack (2002) found that mothers of preterm infants had a greater chance of prolonging lactation beyond 40 weeks corrected age by initiating milk expression at less than six hours following delivery, expressing five or more times per day, practicing kangaroo care, and putting the infant to breast more frequently. Mothers with a longer duration of lactation were able to pump a higher volume of milk early in the pumping experience, making early pumped milk volume a marker for continued milk expression and ultimately prolonging breastfeeding.

The amount and rate of milk that a mother expresses each time she pumps is highly variable among mothers and depends on a number of factors, such as the individual rate of milk production, the vacuum pattern generated by the pump (Mitoulas, Lai, Gurrin, Larsson, & Hartmann, 2002a), and the amount of milk stored in the breast when the mother begins a pumping session. Mitoulas and colleagues (2002b) found that the rate of milk expression changed over the first five-minute expression period, with the rate of milk removal remaining constant over the first 2.5 minutes, but decreasing by five minutes. Prime et al. (2011) identified four patterns of milk ejection in mothers pumping their milk using the Symphony electric breast pump (Medela). The researchers defined milk ejections that had a clearly defined beginning and end as discrete and milk ejections without clear definition were defined as non-discrete.

- Pattern 1 was discrete, with less than five milk ejections over a 15-minute milk expression session.

- Pattern 2 was discrete, with more than five milk ejections.

- Pattern 3 was non-discrete, with five or more milk ejections.

- Pattern 4 was pulsatile, with multiple clearly defined milk ejections occurring with rhythmic repetition.

All patterns removed a similar percentage of available milk. Pattern 4 took longer to remove 80% of the total expression volume than the other patterns. Pattern 1 mothers had less available milk, a lower number of milk ejections, and a lower total volume of expressed milk. The average interval between milk ejections was two minutes. These variations partially explain how mothers with continuous milk flow and large, late milk ejections could take longer than eight minutes to express most of the available milk in the breast, while mothers with other milk ejection patterns can express most of their milk in a shorter period of time.

There is a significant decline in the rate at which milk is removed after the initial milk ejection (Ramsay et al., 2005). Women in this study with the highest increase in ductal diameter during pumping and with more and longer milk ejections expressed more milk. This may help further explain why some mothers are able to express large amounts of milk in short periods of time, and others whose anatomy consists of smaller ducts that do not dilate to a great extent and who do not experience as many let downs during pumping may express lesser amounts of milk at a pumping session.

Mothers should be helped to understand that slower pumping rates or smaller amounts of milk pumped during a pumping session do not always mean they have deficient milk production. These mothers may either need to pump more frequently or be assisted to pump more effectively. Recognizing the milk ejection pattern of a mother may help better tailor milk expression guidance.

Mothers and clinicians are always interested in methods to increase milk volume when pumping. Fewtrell, Loh, Blake, Ridout, & Hawdon (2006) performed a study that looked at the use of nasal oxytocin prior to pumping by preterm mothers and the resulting milk output. Mothers were randomized to either use the oxytocin spray or a placebo while pumping with an Ameda Elite electric breast pump. Mothers used the spray two to five minutes before pumping. The oxytocin group produced more milk over the first two days, with the placebo group matching and exceeding the volume of the oxytocin group by day 5. Many mothers reported a drop in milk output when they stopped using the spray, even though a few of the mothers were actually using the placebo.

Combining milk expression techniques may result in greater milk output as shown by Morton et al. (2009). These researchers demonstrated that in pump-dependent preterm mothers, those that used hand expression greater than five times per day, as well as using an electric pump five times per day during the first three days postpartum produced significantly larger volumes of milk than mothers who only used an electric pump. Furthermore, massaging each breast while using an electric breast pump significantly increased the amount of milk pumped at each session. Over the course of the eight-week study, mothers that combined early hand expression of colostrum in the first three days following birth and who used breast massage and compression while pumping and hand expression, if needed, produced more milk than term mothers (average 955 mL per day). This was independent of pumping frequency in mothers who frequently used hand expression.

The increased volume might be related to the high levels of oxytocin that occur during breast massage (Yokoyama, Ueda, Irahara, & Aono, 1994). This study illustrated that hand expression of colostrum increases milk production in the first two weeks and longer depending on the frequency of use during the first three days. Once mature milk came in, mothers who used breast massage/compression/hand expression in addition to pumping were most likely removing a greater percentage of milk per expression, which allowed greater milk production with less frequent expression. The authors found that the use of high frequency pumping (> seven times per day) was more important for the establishment of lactation than its maintenance. Some mothers in the study who used the hand techniques concurrently with the breast pump were able to maintain and increase milk volume despite less frequent pumping.

Beyond an individually determined number of pumping sessions, increased frequency or duration of pumping may be less effective than better emptying of the breast. Breast massage also changes the pressure gradient between the breast and the pump's collection container. Fluid moves from an area of positive high pressure (created by the letdown reflex and breast massage) to an area of negative low pressure (created by the vacuum in a baby's mouth or generated by a pump). Breast massage increases the positive pressure within the breast, helping milk flow more efficiently. Mothers using a combination of electric pumping and hand expression/breast massage and compression also produced calorie-dense, fat-rich milk that averaged 26 calories per ounce, especially important when feeding preterm infants (Morton et al., 2012).

Increasing the frequency of pumping beyond a certain number of times or lengthening the duration of pumping sessions may be less effective than increasing the degree of emptying of the breast. Daly et al. (1992) showed that the degree of fullness of the breast and the short-term rate of milk synthesis (between feeds) are inversely related; that is, the emptier the breast, the higher the rate of milk synthesis. If a breast is emptied to a greater degree at a breastfeed (or pumping session) than at the previous breastfeed (or pumping session), the rate of milk synthesis will increase, whereas if the breast is emptied to a lesser degree, the rate of milk synthesis after that breastfeed will decrease (Daly, Kent, Owens, & Hartmann, 1996).

Dewey and Lonnerdal (1986) observed that when mothers expressed milk following each breastfeed for two weeks, their milk production increased by an average of 124 mL/24 hours (4 ounces) above their infants' breastmilk intake. Mothers should aim for more complete emptying of the breast each time they hand express and/or pump by making sure that each quadrant of the breast is thoroughly massaged while pumping.

The timing of when breastmilk expression is begun relative to delivery can have an important influence on pumped milk volume. Parker, Sullivan, Krueger, Kelechi & Mueller (2012) studied the effects of early initiation of milk expression on the onset of lactogenesis stage II and milk volume in mothers of very low birthweight infants. Twenty women were randomized to initiate milk expression within 60 minutes of birth (group one) or one to six hours following delivery (group two). Milk volume and timing of lactogenesis stage II was compared between the two groups. Group one produced significantly more milk than group two during the first seven days and at week 3. Group one also demonstrated a significantly earlier lactogenesis stage II. Clinicians may wish to recommend that mothers of preterm or ill infants start milk expression within an hour of birth if possible when the infant cannot be put to breast during that time.

Flaherman et al. (2012) conducted a randomized controlled trial comparing the effect of breast pumping to that of hand expression for mothers of healthy term infants 12 to 36 hours old who were not latching well or not sucking well when latched. Mothers in the hand expression group were more likely to be breastfeeding at two months than mothers assigned to the pump group. Expressed amounts of colostrum were small in both groups (0 to 5 mL in the hand expression group and 0 to 3 mL in the pump group), but could have appeared extremely small and discouraging to mothers using a breast pump. Colostrum often sticks to the sides of the collection kit and bottle and can be difficult to retrieve for feeding to the infant. All of the colostrum that is hand expressed into a plastic spoon or small medicine cup is immediately available to the infant.

Ohyama et al. (2010) found that manual expression yielded twice as much colostrum as did electric pumping during the first 48 hours following delivery in mothers who delivered between 29 and 39 weeks. Net milk yield was 2 mL (range 0 to 12.6 mL) in the hand expression group and 0.6 mL (range 0 to 7.2 mL) in the pump group. Mothers in this study alternated between manual expression and using a double electric pump every three hours, such that every other expression session was done by hand.

The warming of tissues is a known therapeutic intervention that has the effect of increasing local blood flow and metabolism in tissues, facilitating excretion of tissue waste materials and phagocytosis, and enhancing tissue nutrition (Barret et al., 2010). Warm compresses placed on the breasts have long been recommended to aid the let down reflex. Kent, Geddes, Hepworth, & Hartmann (2011) found that warmed pump flanges resulted in a larger amount of available milk removal. Yigit et al. (2012) studied whether warming the breast prior to pumping would increase the volume of milk expressed from a warmed breast compared with the contralateral breast which was not warmed. Mothers placed a warm compress (40.5C/104.9F) on one breast prior to pumping with an electric breast pump. The amount of milk obtained from the warmed breasts was significantly higher than that obtained from the non-warmed breasts. Warming probably has an enhancing effect on the milk ducts or milk flow, allowing more milk to be pumped, rather than increasing actual breastmilk production.

Many of these studies show that mothers who possess risk factors for underproduction of milk (preterm, late preterm, cesarean, separation, non-latching, ill infant) can greatly benefit from early initiation of expressing (within the first hour of birth for mothers separated from their infant) and from using hand expression in conjunction with the use of breast pumps to decrease the risk of insufficient milk. The availability of more colostrum and breastmilk reduces the likelihood of formula supplementation and continued falling milk production. With insufficient milk, the most common reason for premature weaning, interventions that hold promise for preventing this problem to begin with should be included in feeding plans when possible.

If pumping more times does not improve milk output, and/or the mother cannot pump more times during the day or week, suggest that she pump more effectively. This can be done by:

- Eliciting the milk ejection reflex prior to pumping. Some mothers find the use of oxytocin nasal spray helpful in eliciting the milk-ejection reflex. While it may not increase overall volume of milk pumped (Fewtrell et al., 2006), its use may help individual mothers overcome delayed milk ejection and reduce pumping time. Oxytocin nasal spray is no longer available as a packaged nasal spray, but can be obtained by prescription from a compounding pharmacy. The original preparation,

Syntocinon, contained 40 units/mL. The current prescription is written for a 15 mL nasal spray using standard oxytocin. The dosage is one to two sprays in the nares, followed by breastfeeding in one to two minutes (Lawrence & Lawrence, 2011).

- Massaging each quadrant of the breast while pumping to help drain the breast as thoroughly as possible.

- Expressing milk following each breastfeeding of the infant.

- Warming the pump flange and the breasts prior to pumping.

- Checking that the flange is not too small.

- Changing to a different pump. This sometimes helps increase milk expression. Different suction curves may provide a better fit between mother and pump.

Chapter 13.
Scenarios and Pumping Plans

Given what is known about pumps and techniques to make pumping more effective, the following scenarios with suggested pumping plans may offer the clinician another resource for helping mothers who must use a breast pump.

Employed Mothers

The first 14 days postpartum are a window of time that is critical to the calibration of the milk supply and the continuation of breastfeeding beyond two weeks. It is notable that in preterm mothers, the amount of milk produced at 10–14 days is predictive of milk volumes and continuance of lactation at three, four, and five weeks postpartum (Hill et al., 1999). Mothers who intend to return to employment should be advised to exclusively breastfeed eight to 12 times each 24 hours and work toward an abundant milk supply. Breastfeeding problems should be addressed and remedied as quickly as possible. Based on how old the infant will be when the mother returns to employment, the mother and clinician can construct a breastfeeding plan for her maternity leave and after employment resumes (Biagioli, 2003).

Mothers will need differing guidance based on the age of the infant when returning to work. Mothers returning to work when the baby will be six months old may find that expressing milk once or twice each workday meets the breastmilk needs of the infant and maintains good milk production because infants usually start solid foods around this age.

Mothers with a three-month maternity leave will need to have breastfeeding well established, have worked through any early breastfeeding problems, and have an infant gaining weight appropriately. She may want to consider pumping milk several times per week prior to the return to employment to have a milk reserve in the freezer for times of fluctuating milk supply. Mothers can pump this milk after feedings or in between feedings, whichever gives the best results. Milk can be stored and/or frozen in amounts that the baby typically takes at a feeding. Mothers should avoid storing large amounts of milk in a bottle to avoid wasting milk if the baby does not consume the entire amount. Mothers will generally need to pump milk at work about two to three times, depending on the length of the workday, her infant's needs, and her own comfort.

Mothers who can take only a two, four, or six week break from work or school present a more complex situation. It is especially important that early breastfeeding problems be resolved before the mother returns to work or school. Breastfeeding management for these mothers may be somewhat different than for mothers with a longer maternity leave. Dwindling milk production and/or insufficient milk supply are often pressing problems if a mother starts back to work so soon after giving birth. If a mother cannot express sufficient amounts of milk for her infant or if she does not have an abundant milk supply at the time of her return to work, she often begins supplementing with formula, contributing to a further decrease in milk production.

A potential preventive approach to this very early return to work scenario is to use the model of initiating and maintaining abundant milk production in the preterm mother. This model recommends achieving a high milk production by 10–14 days postpartum, such that the mother is producing 50% more milk than the infant actually needs (Hill et al., 1999). This extent of overproduction increases milk production quickly and serves as a buffer to compensate for any milk volume decrease when the mother starts back to work or school, a situation that is not an uncommon side effect of an early return to work. This excess milk is frozen and can be used on the first day back to work or school and anytime the mother experiences a fluctuation in the amount of milk she pumps while separated from the infant.

To achieve a 50% overproduction or to at least produce more milk than the baby requires, mothers will need to hand express and/or pump milk several times each day in addition to nursing the baby. A method for achieving high milk output was suggested by Morton and colleagues (2009) who demonstrated that in pump-dependent preterm mothers, those that used hand expression greater than five times per day, as well as using an electric pump five times per day during the first three days postpartum produced significantly larger volumes of milk than mothers who only used an electric pump. Furthermore, massaging each breast while using an electric breast pump significantly increased the amount of milk pumped at each session.

Dewey and Lonnerdal (1986) observed that when mothers expressed milk following each breastfeed for two weeks, their milk production increased by an average of 124 mL/24 hours (4 ounces) above their infants' breastmilk intake. Mothers should aim for more complete emptying of the breast each time they hand express and/or pump by making sure that each quadrant of the breast is thoroughly massaged while pumping. Applying the above knowledge and techniques to a mother returning to work in the early weeks following birth might generate a plan similar to the one in Box 13.1. Mothers can aim to come as close as possible to this plan.

Box 13.1. Sample Pumping Plan for a Mother Returning to Work or School Two to Six Weeks Postpartum

- During the first three days following birth, aim to breastfeed the infant approximately eight or more times each 24 hours. Additionally, hand express milk five times each day.

- After the first three days and during the time prior to returning to work or school, hand express or pump milk following as many breastfeedings as possible. If a pump is used, massage and compress each quadrant of each breast during each pumping session. For mothers returning to work at six weeks, even starting to pump at four weeks in most situations should be sufficient to preserve an abundant milk supply unless any breastfeeding problems remain unresolved.

- Obtain a personal-use (or rental hospital-grade multi-user pump) double electric breast pump.

- Store the expressed milk in the freezer, labeling it with the date it was expressed, so the oldest can be used first.

- Pump or hand express milk once during any long gaps between the infant's feedings.

- Aim to drain the breasts as thoroughly as possible.

- A bottle can be introduced at seven days if returning to work or school at two weeks; at three weeks if returning to work or school at four weeks; and at five weeks if returning to work or school at six weeks.

Source: Walker, M. Breastfeeding and employment: making it work. Amarillo, TX: Hale Publishing, 2011

Mothers want a moderate oversupply, but not so much as to cause leaking, pain, plugged ducts, or mastitis. Mothers returning to work at three months or later have much more leeway in when to start pumping for a stash in the freezer and a small oversupply to account for a potential drop in production right after the return to work. These mothers will not need to start pumping until a couple of weeks before their planned return to work.

Time is in short supply for employed breastfeeding mothers. Clinicians can provide the following time-saving ideas for pumping at work (Walker, 2011):

• Listen to the sounds of the baby by recording them. Mothers can make a slide show with photos and sounds of their baby recorded on an iPhone, iPod, mp3 player, Smartphone, or other electronic device used with ear buds (Roche-Paull, 2010). This provides a relaxed atmosphere and a mechanism to condition the letdown reflex.

• Elicit the milk ejection reflex prior to pumping by using reverse pressure softening, massaging the breasts, or using photos or sounds of the baby. This helps reduce pumping time as pumps can take up to two minutes to achieve milk ejection.

• Use mental imagery or one of the baby's blankets to facilitate letdown.

• Massage and compress each quadrant of the breast while pumping.

• Use of a hands-free bra allows mothers to continue working while pumping if the mother has an office type of job and dedicated pumping space.

• Have two or three pump collection kits for use during their work time. The kits can be cleaned at home instead of having to wash pump collection parts after each use. For mothers who have access to refrigeration, the pump collection parts can be rinsed or cleaned with a sanitizing wipe and placed in a zip lock bag in a refrigerator between uses, and then thoroughly cleaned at home. If the mother has access to a microwave, she can place pump parts in a bag made especially for sterilizing breast pump parts and microwave the collection kit between uses.

• Use sanitizing wipes to quickly clean pump parts if the mother does not have access to running water.

• Pump directly into the bottles that will be used the next day. This eliminates having to transfer milk into other containers.

• Keep nursing pads at work to avoid stains on clothing, especially if the mother is in long meetings or has a long duty assignment that takes her past the regular time she would be pumping. Some mothers keep a change of clothing in their bag, just in case.

Finding a time and place to pump is not always easy, especially if a mother has a non-traditional job or does not work in an office-like setting. Mothers have worked out clever and original pumping accommodations with their employer. Spaces to pump need to be no larger than 4 feet by 5 feet and do not need to be permanent structures. The US Department of Health and Human Services Office on Women's Health (OWH) is creating an online searchable resource to showcase creative solutions for supporting employees who are nursing their babies. The resource will be available in Fall 2012.

Mothers of Preterm, Late Preterm, Ill Infants, or Infants With Conditions That Preclude Feeding at the Breast Who Will Be Pump Dependent

For mothers of preterm and late preterm infants or infants unable to feed directly from the breast, initiation and protection of the maternal milk supply starts in the hospital. If the baby is unable to transfer colostrum, then hand expression or pumping should be started within one hour of delivery (Parker et al., 2012) or at the latest by six hours of delivery (Hill, Aldag, & Chatterton, 2001). Anecdotal reports describe some mothers as having a considerable colostrum bolus available by pump immediately following delivery. Combining milk expression techniques may result in greater milk output as shown by Morton et al. (2009). Hand expression five times per day, as well as using an electric pump eight times per day during the first three days postpartum should be recommended. Mothers should obtain and use a high quality hospital-grade multi-user breast pump. Most mothers will need to pump until the infant reaches 40–42 weeks post-menstrual age or sometimes longer. Preterm infants usually do not drain the breasts well enough for the mother to stop pumping until the infant's due date has been reached.

Milk production should be watched very carefully during the first 14 days following delivery, as there is a high potential for insufficient milk (Hill, Aldag, Chatterton, & Zinaman, 2005). Mothers who are exclusively or predominantly pumping should target a minimal output of 3500 mL/week (118 oz) or 500 ml/day (17 oz) by the end of the second week to achieve optimal output for sustained lactation (Hill et al., 1999). The optimal volume of milk by 10–14 days postpartum is >750mL/24 hours (25 oz), with outputs of <350mL/24 hours (12 oz) placing the milk supply at an extremely high risk of remaining insufficient (Hurst & Meier, 2010). Milk volumes that reach 800–1000mL/24 hours (27 oz - 34 oz) by 10–14 days provides a reserve such that if the maternal milk supply drops by as much as 50% during the infant's hospitalization, sufficient volume will remain to adequately nourish her infant upon discharge from the hospital (Hurst & Meier, 2010). Mothers of twins should target a minimum of 1000mL/24 hours (34 oz) of pumped milk, assuming that 500 mL/day (17 oz) is the minimum for singleton infants. Mothers should keep pumping logs that include 24-hour milk output, so faltering milk production can be addressed immediately. Once lactogenesis II has occurred and mature milk has come in, mothers should add breast massage and compression to frequent pumping. Mothers should use the maximum comfortable vacuum of the pump. When milk flow stops, mothers should then stop pumping, massage the breasts briefly for one to two minutes and attempt to remove the remaining milk as best they can by either hand expressing or resuming double pumping or single pumping of each breast, whichever works best (Morton et al., 2009). Hand expression and breast massage techniques are demonstrated at http://newborns.stanford.edu/Breastfeeding/ (see "Hand Expressing Milk" and "Maximizing Milk Production"). Both clinicians and mothers can view these videos to learn the techniques. There are no specific time parameters for each pumping session. Specifying a time frame for pumping may be less effective than providing instructions for more effective pumping. Pumping durations can range from 10 to 45 minutes and are highly individual. Some mothers find that small incentives can help them engage in the necessary frequency of pumping, which can be time consuming and require the mother to structure her day around pumping. Clinicians have recommended that mothers set out seven or eight little treats and consume one each time she pumps. Some mothers find the use of oxytocin nasal spray helpful in eliciting the milk-ejection reflex. While it may not increase the overall volume of milk pumped (Fewtrell et al., 2006), its use may help individual mothers overcome delayed milk ejection and reduce pumping time. This may be helpful in times of increased stress or if the infant experiences medical problems when mothers may experience a delay in milk ejection. Box 13.2 provides a sample pumping plan for preterm mothers.

Box 13.2. Sample Pumping Plan for a Pump Dependent Mother

- Begin pumping/hand expressing in the hospital within one hour of birth and no later than six hours following delivery.

- Double pump eight times per day and hand express five times per day for the first three postpartum days.

- Obtain a hospital-grade, multi-user double electric breast pump for use at home.

- Use the proper size flanges. Obtain a larger size if: pain is experienced while pumping, the nipple rubs against the side of the nipple tunnel or sticks to the side, the nipple does not move freely in the tunnel after about five minutes of pumping, the entire nipple does not fit into the nipple tunnel, the nipple does not move back and forth in a smooth rhythmical motion, the tip of the nipple becomes sore or blistered, there are areas of the breast that are not well drained after pumping, a ring of sloughed skin or specks of skin are seen on the inside of the shield after pumping, the base of the nipple is blanching (turning white) while pumping, or there is minimal or no areolar tissue being pulled into the tunnel of the flange.

- Pump eight times per day using the maximum comfortable vacuum after the milk comes in. The number of times pumped each day may decrease over time based on achieving a full milk supply in the early days and weeks.

- Double pump both breasts, and simultaneously massage and compress each breast.

- Stop pumping and massage each breast for one to two minutes when the milk flow stops, then either resume pumping or hand express as much of the remaining milk as possible.

- Keep a pumping log of milk output and aim for 750 mL/day (25 oz) of expressed milk by 10 to 14 days postpartum.

- Elicit the milk ejection first before using the pump to decrease pumping time.

- Try oxytocin nasal spray if the milk ejection is delayed.

Mothers of Late Preterm Infants (34–37 Weeks) Who Are Not Completely Pump Dependent

Mothers of late preterm infants who are not completely pump dependent may also need to express milk until their baby is fully established at breast. Even though many late preterm infants can feed at the breast, it is often done so in a relatively ineffective manner.

Late preterm infants are at a disadvantage in terms of feeding skills. They are born with low energy stores (both subcutaneous and brown fat). They have high-energy demands, poor feeding abilities, and are sleepy, with fewer and shorter awake periods. They tire easily when feeding, have a weak suck and low tone, demonstrate an inability to sustain sucking, and may have a small mouth, with uncoordinated oral-motor movements. They are easily over-stimulated and may shut down before consuming adequate amounts of colostrum or milk. They may take only small volumes of milk during the early days in the hospital, which are often sufficient for that period of time, but exhibit feeding difficulties when higher volumes of milk intake become necessary for normal growth. While some babies may demonstrate adequate muscle tone initially, this tone may be rapidly depleted during a feeding, indicating decreased endurance. Postural stability may be immature, creating a less efficient feeding pattern. Late preterm infants experience reduced tone in the muscles involved with feeding, which coupled with neurologic immaturity of the suck, swallow, breathe cycle results in uncoordinated and ineffective milk intake at the breast. If treated like a normal term newborn, they are at an increased risk for inadequate nourishment. They may go through the motions of feeding, but may transfer little, if any, milk for their efforts (Walker, 2009). This increases the risk of inadequate milk production and raises the necessity for monitoring milk production more closely.

In order to compensate for the infant's feeding immaturity, many mothers will need to pump their milk after feedings and/or in between feedings to assure adequate production. Mothers may need to pump milk for the first two weeks until the infant is completely established at breast and gaining weight well. Most mothers will need to pump until the infant reaches 40–42 weeks post-menstrual age, as late preterm infants usually do not drain the breasts well enough for the mother to stop pumping until the infant's due date has been reached. Mothers can wean from pumping by dropping one pumping per day per week until she either discontinues completely. She may wish to continue pumping one to two times a day for storage if she is returning to work or wants to have extra milk on hand for separations.

Chapter 14. Problems With Pumps and Pumping

There are a number of common problems seen with pumps and pumping scenarios. No matter why a mother is pumping, a low or diminishing milk supply ranks as a prime concern and problem. Clinicians who see mothers in the hospital are in a prime position to reduce the likelihood of insufficient milk production in many mothers who are at a high risk for this condition by providing guidelines discussed in the previous chapters. Other clinicians will meet the mother who is already encountering milk supply issues.

Diminished Milk Production

Low milk supply issues are extremely worrisome to mothers and one of the most common problems that mothers who are regularly expressing breastmilk encounter. It is important to identify the etiology of the problem and create a workable solution as quickly as possible. Mothers may complain that they are pumping less milk at work or that their infant is consuming more milk than they can pump. Pump-dependent mothers may notice diminishing or erratic amounts of pumped milk. Some mothers may have a chronic milk supply issue and need guidance for interventions they can try. Other mothers may simply pump less milk over time or only be able to pump small amounts of milk from the start. Contributors to low milk production or only being able to pump small amounts of milk, along with possible solutions, are offered below:

Pumping Schedule

If the mother is employed, ask if anything has changed regarding how many times the mother pumps each day, where she pumps, if she has been traveling, if her pumping breaks are shorter, if the breaks are erratic, if her working hours have changed, or if pumping breaks have been skipped. Changes like this may reduce milk output temporarily, and if not addressed, they may result in a permanent reduction of the milk supply.

Can the mother remedy this at the work site by pumping more times for shorter periods? Can she nurse the baby when she drops off the baby with the childcare provider? Can she arrive at work a little earlier and pump first thing before starting her workday? Can she add another pumping session right before she goes to bed? Can she add several extra pumping sessions on her days off?

Pumping every 45–120 minutes for several periods of time during the day is called "power pumping," "cluster pumping," or "super pumping." A modification of this can be suggested whereby a mother pumps for as long as it takes to elicit the first milk ejection reflex and removes the milk made available during the time the milk ducts stay dilated. Up to 45% of the milk available in the breast is released during the first milk letdown (Ramsey et al., 2006). This may take no longer than five minutes. The mother can pump again in 15 minutes or so to once again take advantage of the first and largest milk ejection reflex during a pumping session. She may repeat this pattern for an hour several times a day when she has time or during her days off.

Mothers who work rotating shifts or have erratic opportunities for pumping, such as mothers in the military (Roche-Paull (2010), may find it especially difficult to find the time and place to pump as many times as necessary to keep up good milk production. Mothers may need to get creative in how they handle pumping. Many mothers are fearful and embarrassed to talk with their supervisor about their pumping needs. A letter from the infant's healthcare provider describing that breastmilk has been prescribed for the infant and that the physician requests time be made available for pumping at work may help.[29]

Pumping More Effectively

If pumping more times does not improve milk output and/or the mother cannot pump more times during the day or week, suggest that she pump more effectively. This can be done by:

- Eliciting the milk ejection reflex prior to pumping. Some mothers find the use of oxytocin nasal spray helpful in eliciting the milk-ejection reflex.

- Massaging each quadrant of the breast while pumping to help drain the breast as thoroughly as possible.

- Expressing milk following each breastfeeding of the infant.

- Arranging for pumping sessions closer together.

- Power pumping twice per day.

---

29 http://www.dshs.state.tx.us/wichd/bf/bfphyletter.shtm and http://massbreastfeeding.org/pdf/doctorletter.pdf

- Warming the flanges before pumping.

- Advising that when milk flow stops to turn off the pump, massage and compress the breasts, and either start pumping again or hand express residual milk.

Pump Mechanics

Fluctuating or reduced milk production may sometimes be attributed to issues with the pump itself or how it is being used. Check the following to make sure the pump is working efficiently.

- Check that the settings are adjusted for maximal milk output. Pump settings can be varied on most of the electric pumps. Both the cycling characteristics and amount of vacuum can be adjusted for comfort, as well as for efficiency.

- Check that the mother is using the maximum amount of vacuum she is comfortable with (Kent et al., 2008).

- Check the motor with a pressure gauge, especially if the mother complains of a gradual decrease in the amount of milk she pumps at each pumping session. The motor may be worn down or need adjusting. If the pump vacuum is suboptimal and it is a rental pump or hospital-grade pump, it should be returned to the manufacturer for adjustment. The mother will need another pump.

- Check the batteries if the pump is battery operated. It may need new batteries, even though it may still be running. Rechargeable batteries may not be as effective as regular or lithium batteries.

- Check the fit of the flange. An improperly fitting flange may impede milk flow. If the nipple shows little movement in the flange, if there are flakes of skin left on the flange after pumping, if the nipple is discolored while pumping, if the junction of the nipple and areola blanches while pumping, or if there is nipple pain, the mother may need a larger flange. Unusually shaped breasts may not fit in standard flanges preventing a good seal between flange and breast. The mother can try a soft flange insert, which may help to provide a better fit between flange and breast.

- Check that all parts of the collection kit are assembled correctly and that there are no leaks, cracks, holes, or tears in the tubing.

- Check any membranes or barrier filters to be sure they are not ripped, wet, worn out, defective, or dirty and that they are attached correctly. If there is a problem with the barrier filter, it will need to be replaced.

- Have the mother check that the pump is not overheating from blocked air vents or from being placed on a soft surface while running.

- Have the mother try a different pump if these suggestions do not work to increase milk production. A different suction curve may provide a boost to milk output.

- Check the mother's expectations of the pump. The mother may think a small electric pump should behave in the same manner as a hospital-grade, multi-user pump. The small pump may be working correctly based on its capabilities, but not in an effective enough manner to support an abundant milk supply.

Maternal Health Issues

Clinicians should check to see if mothers are taking any medication that could depress milk production, such as pseudoephedrine (Sudafed). Aljazaf et al. (2003) found that this decongestant reduced milk production by 24% with one 60 mg dose. Mothers with poor or marginal milk production should probably avoid this medication. Decongestant nasal sprays are a better option for nursing mothers, as they do not affect milk production.

Has the mother started birth control pills or have her menstrual cycles returned? Starting combined birth control pills prior to six weeks postpartum should be avoided due to the possibility of reducing milk production (Jackson, 2011). Some mothers report a drop in their milk supply just prior to or during their menstrual periods. Anecdotal recommendations from clinicians have suggested that the mother take a daily dose of 500 to 1,000 mg of a calcium/magnesium supplement from midcycle (ovulation) through the first three days of her period to avoid supply fluctuations (West & Marasco, 2009).

Check if the mother has been ill, is eating poorly, has polycystic ovarian syndrome (Marasco, Marmet, & Shell, 2000), is experiencing anemia (Henly et al., 1995) or is hypothyroid (Marasco, 2006; Motil et al., 1994). Persistent and stubborn milk supply issues that do not respond to other interventions may have a hormonal or nutritional basis and may benefit from lab work to check iron and thyroid levels. Sometimes, a mother's hectic schedule leaves little time for well-balanced meals. Nutritious snacks may help meet the needs for a balanced diet.

Stress is an enemy of expressing milk. Ask the mother if she has experienced increased stress, assumed additional duties at work or at home, or if anyone in her family is ill or has had a health status change. Since stress can impede milk production (Lau, 2001), as well as the milk ejection reflex, the sources of stress should be discovered and measures taken to reduce it.

Overfeeding By Childcare Providers

Some mothers may assume that their milk production is dropping when their infant starts consuming more and more milk at childcare. If mothers cannot keep up with this increasing demand, they interpret this as insufficient milk. Mothers should check with their childcare provider regarding the amount of milk the baby takes at each feeding and if any is being discarded following feedings. If the infant does not finish the bottle, then smaller amounts of milk should be put in each container. Ask the mother to check if the baby is being overfed by being offered a bottle every time he or she fusses. This can make it appear that a mother has a dwindling milk supply or that she cannot keep up with the needs of her infant. Mothers should request that other soothing techniques be used by childcare providers, such as holding, rocking, or wearing the baby in a sling.

Older babies have a range of daily milk intake, with an average of 25 to 30 ounces in a 24-hour period. Depending on her work schedule and the size and age of the baby, mothers might leave about 10–15 ounces with the caregiver each day. More milk might be necessary depending on the number of hours the mother is away from the baby and the baby's appetite. Mothers can have the childcare provider keep one to two bottles of breastmilk in their freezer for growth spurts or unforeseen late pick up. Some mothers are able to breastfeed when they drop off the infant at childcare and again when they pick up the baby. This helps reduce the time during each day that the baby must be fed pumped milk and can result in one less bottle of pumped milk being needed at childcare each day (Berggren, 2006).

Sore Nipples

Mothers whose nipples are already sore should exercise caution when using a breast pump, especially if the nipple is macerated, has an open wound, or is bleeding. Hand expression may be a better option in these situations. To avoid soreness caused by pumping, mothers can:

- Avoid using a pump that cycles less than 40 times per minute. Such a pump holds vacuum on the nipple for prolonged periods of time during each suction phase.

- Use a properly fitting flange that does not restrict nipple movement or strangulate the nipple. Some mothers start out a pumping session with a standard size flange and switch to a larger one midway through as the nipples swell. Mothers may need to change flange sizes during the pumping experience if the nipples become sore from pumping.

- Use a larger flange or a different pump if the nipple turns purple while pumping. This may indicate that the vacuum curve is not allowing venous blood to leave the nipple and is blocking oxygen rich blood from entering. Mothers may need a larger flange or a different pump, with a suction curve better suited to the mother. The Symphony electric pump (Medela) has a more gradual pull and release. The Ameda electric pump has a short push (positive pressure at the end of each cycle) that allows the nipple to re-perfuse.

- Elicit milk ejection prior to the start of pumping to decrease the time vacuum is applied to the breast when milk is not flowing.

- Pump for shorter periods of time, but more frequently.

- Lubricate the flange with a little olive oil.

- Temporarily reduce the amount of vacuum they are using until the nipples feel better.

Chapter 14. Galactogogues

A common intervention for low milk supply is the use of herbal, botanical, dietary, and/or pharmaceutical galactogogues. Herbal and botanical galactogogues have been used for centuries around the world, but research-based evidence is sparse regarding their use, dosage, and effectiveness. Many cultures have special foods that are given to new mothers to encourage abundant milk production. Herbalists, doctors of traditional Chinese medicine, homeopaths, and naturopaths are practitioners whose education and practice include the use of these preparations and who represent a good resource for guidance. Clinicians may wish to consult with an expert if they are not familiar with these preparations, as they come in many forms and dosages, are not standardized, and their effectiveness and safety cannot be guaranteed.

Some mothers will not benefit from the use of these preparations, and others may find that they are quite effective in increasing milk production. There is no way to know whether one preparation will work better than another for a particular mother. There are many herbs, herbal preparations, and homeopathic remedies that various sources recommend for boosting milk production. These include alfalfa (Medicago sativa), aniseed (Pimpinella anisum), blessed thistle (Cnicus benedictus), borage (Borago officinalis), caraway seed (Carum carvi), chasteberry (Vitex agnus-castus), dandelion (Taraxacum officinale), dill seed (Anethum graveolens), fennel (Foeniculum vulgare), fenugreek seed (Trigonella foenum-graecum), goat's rue (Galega officinalis), marshmallow root (Althaea officinalis), milk thistle (Silybum marianum), nettle or stinging nettle (Urtica urens or Urtica dioica), oat straw (Avena sativa), red clover blossoms (Trifolium pratense), red raspberry (Rubus idaeus), saw palmetto (Serenoa repens), shatavari (Asparagus racemosus), and vervain (Verbena officinalis) (West & Marasco, 2009).

The most commonly used herbal galactogogue is fenugreek (Trigonella foenum-graecum). Turkyilmaz and colleagues (2011) studied whether consuming herbal tea containing fenugreek affected milk production and infant weight gain during the early postnatal period, prior to any milk insufficiency problems. They found that the mean measured milk volume in the group consuming fenugreek tea was significantly higher than in the control and placebo groups. Infants in the experimental group also regained their birth weight sooner than those in the placebo and control groups. This study suggests that for mothers returning to work very soon after delivery or perhaps for mothers at an increased risk for milk supply problems, consuming fenugreek tea may be advantageous in contributing to an abundant milk supply during the early weeks postpartum.

DiPierro, Callegari, Carotenuto, and Tapia (2008) took another approach when they studied the effects of a standardized extract from milk thistle (Silybum marianum), called Silymarin, on milk production in 50 mothers with low milk production. Micronized to enhance absorption, Silymarin was given to 25 mothers and a placebo was given to the other 25 mothers for 63 days. At the end of the study, the mothers in the experimental group had an 85.95% increase in milk output compared with a 32.09% increase in the placebo group. This preparation is available commercially in Europe as PiuLatte.[30]

Commercial galactogogue preparations typically combine several of these herbals or botanicals, such as Mother's Milk Blend Tea (chamomile, catnip, fennel, stinging nettle, and lavender), More Milk Plus (a tincture blend of fenugreek, blessed thistle, stinging nettle, and fennel), and Mother's Lactaflow (a tincture blend of fennel, blessed thistle, goat's rue, and fenugreek). Clinicians need to closely follow mothers consuming galactogogues to assure that the preparations are effective and that the mother and baby are not experiencing any undesirable side effects.

Shatavari (Asparagus racemosus) is a popular galactogogue in India and China, but there is little evidence of its effectiveness in increasing milk supplies. One study found that it had no effect on increasing prolactin levels or milk production (Sharma, Ramji, Kumari, & Bapna, 1996).

Recombinant human prolactin (r-hPRL) has been shown to be an effective galactogogue (Page-Wilson, Smith, & Welt, 2007). In one study of mothers with prolactin deficiency and mothers of preterm infants with lactation insufficiency, peak prolactin increased in mothers treated with r-hPRL every 12 hours (Powe et al., 2010).

Another study of mothers with documented prolactin deficiency and mothers with lactation insufficiency that developed while they were pumping breast milk for their preterm infants, found that r-hPRL not only increased milk volume (73 to 146 mL/day; 2.4 to 5 oz), but also enhanced the anti-infective properties of the milk (Powe et al., 2011).

Two of the most commonly used pharmaceutical galactogogues are metoclopramide (Reglan) and domperidone (Motilium). Metoclopramide is primarily used for treating reflux in patients with low gastric tone.

---

30 http://www.farmamica.com/store/dettview1_l2.php?id=3407

Metoclopramide also has the effect of stimulating prolactin release from the pituitary and increasing milk production in mothers with low milk supply. Doses of 30–45 mg/day appear most effective. It is important to note that not all mothers will respond with increased milk production if their prolactin levels are already normal. Clinicians need to exercise some caution with this medication because it crosses the blood-brain barrier and may cause central nervous system side effects, such as involuntary body movements and depression. Mothers with depression or a history of depression may not be suitable candidates for this medication. Some authors, however, have considered metoclopramide compatible with breastfeeding, as long as its dose does not exceed 45 mg/day (Zuppa et al., 2010).

Domperidone, a potent dopamine D2 receptor antagonist, is approved only for the treatment of gastroparesis, nausea, and vomiting in most countries, but it can be purchased over the counter for use in situations of milk insufficiency, except in the United States. In the United States, domperidone is classified as an orphan drug that has not yet received clearance from the Food and Drug Administration (FDA) for use in breastfeeding mothers with milk insufficiency. It does not readily cross the blood-brain barrier and rarely causes extrapyramidal adverse reactions, which makes it a better choice for milk enhancement than metoclopramide. A study by Wan et al. (2008) found domperidone to be an effective galactogogue for most, but not all mothers, with side-effects of dry mouth, abdominal cramping, and headache noted in some mothers. Jantarasaengaram & Sreewapa (2011) found that postpartum treatment with domperidone can augment breastmilk production in mothers after a full-term cesarean section, with minimal adverse effects. Mothers undergoing a cesarean section for a full-term infant who received domperidone produced significantly more milk on days one through four than mothers in the control group. Domperidone may not further enhance milk production in mothers with an already high prolactin level. Mothers in the United States may often be able to obtain this medication from compounding pharmacies.

For over a thousand years, acupuncture has been used in China as an effective treatment for insufficient milk (Zhao & Guo, 2006; Jenner & Filshie, 2002). A study by Clavey (1996) discussed acupuncture as an effective remedy for milk insufficiency, with over a 90% effectiveness rate when acupuncture was initiated within 20 days of birth, but less than an 85% success rate after 20 days postpartum. The earlier postpartum the treatment was begun, the quicker the results and the more likely that milk production significantly improved. However, acupuncture was not as effective if the mother had poor breast development. Wei, Wang, Han, & Li (2008) described the very effective use of electroacupuncture at the point of the body identified as Shaoze (SI 1) in 46 mothers with insufficient milk. Neri and colleagues (2011) conducted a study to investigate the effect of acupuncture treatment in the maintenance of exclusive breastfeeding during the first three months postpartum. Exclusive breastfeeding at three months was significantly higher in mothers who had been treated with acupuncture. While not widely used for milk insufficiency in the United States, acupuncture may hold some promise for some mothers when other forms of treatment are not well tolerated or are ineffective.

Another form of traditional Chinese medicine that has been used to treat low milk production in mothers experiencing a cesarean section is auricular points sticking-pressure. Auricular therapy/pressure is similar to acupressure. Pressure is applied to specific locations on the ear using natural seeds, a blunt-headed stick, or fingertips. The outer ear has about 200 of these acupoints, where pressure can be applied to treat numerous diseases and conditions. Zhou and colleagues (2009) conducted a study on 116 post-cesarean mothers, looking at the volume of milk produced, the use of supplementary feedings, and the serum prolactin levels in the experimental and control group. Mothers treated with auricular points sticking-pressure therapy showed elevated milk volumes, lower levels of supplementary feedings, and higher prolactin levels than mothers in the control group. Mothers should always seek qualified and experienced practitioners of these alternative forms of treatments.

Conclusion

No breast pump is perfect for all mothers and all situations. Clinicians use their best judgment, clinical experience, and available evidence to help mothers find the right pump for the mother's needs. Various features of pumps change constantly, with clinicians needing to be aware of such changes and ready to adjust recommendations accordingly.

Breast pumps are not needed by every mother. But when they are needed, there are a variety of pumps from which to choose. Mothers benefit from guidance on how to use and care for the pump, as well as the receipt of an individualized evidence-based pumping plan created to preserve and protect an abundant milk supply.

Resources

Pump Manufacturers

Ameda
475 Half Day Rd
Lincolnshire, IL 60069
1–866–99-AMEDA
www.Ameda.com

Bailey Medical
2216 Sunset Drive
Los Osos, CA 93402
1–800–413–3216
www.baileymed.com/

Hygeia II Medical Group, Inc.
1600 East Orangethorpe Ave.
Fullerton, CA 92831
1- 888-PUMP–4-MOM (888–786–7466)
or 714–515–7571
www.hygeiababy.com

Lansinoh Laboratories, Inc.
333 North Fairfax Street, Suite 400
Alexandria, VA 22314
1- 800–292–4794
www.lansinoh.com/

Limerick, Inc.
2150 N. Glenoaks Blvd.
Burbank, CA 91504–4327
1- 877-limeric (546–3742)
www.limerickinc.com

Medela, Inc. - Breastfeeding
P.O. Box 660
1101 Corporate Drive
McHenry, IL. 60050 / USA
1–800 435 8316
www.medelabreastfeedingus.com

Philips Avent
P.O. Box 77900
1070 MX Amsterdam
The Netherlands

1–800–542–8368
www.usa.philips.com

Playtex Baby
Energizer Personal Care
890 Mountain Ave.
New Providence, NJ 07974
1–888–310–4290
www.playtexbaby.com

The First Years
1111 W. 22ⁿᵈ St. Suite 320
Oak Brook, IL 60523
1–800–704–8697
www.thefirstyears.com/wps/portal/

Use Of Herbals And Botanicals For Insufficient Milk Production

Rister, R., Klein, S., & Riggins, C. (1998). *The complete German Commission E Monographs: Therapeutic guide to herbal medicines* (1ˢᵗ ed.). Austin TX: American Botanical Council.

Humphrey, S. (2003). *The nursing mother's herbal.* Minneapolis, MN: Fairview Press.

Low Dog, T. (2005). *Women's health in complementary and integrative medicine: clinical guide.* St. Louis, MO: Elsevier, Churchill, Livingstone.

Thomson Healthcare. (2007). *PDR for herbal medicines* (4ᵗʰ ed.). Montvale, NJ: Thomson Reuters.

Jacobson, H. (2004). *Mother food for breastfeeding mothers.* Otsego, MI: Pagefree Publishing.

West, D., & Marasco, L. (2009). *The breastfeeding mother's guide to making more milk.* New York: McGraw Hill.

Books

Casemore, S. (2004). Exclusively pumping breast milk: a guide to providing expressed breast milk for your baby. Napanee, Ontario, Canada: Gray Lion Publishing. http://www.exclusivelypumping.com/

Stafford, S. (2003). *Pumping breast milk successfully.* New York, NY: iUniverse.

Walker, M. (2011). *Breastfeeding and employment.* Amarillo, TX: Hale Publishing.

Watson Genna, C. (2009). *Selecting and using breastfeeding tools.* Amarillo, TX: Hale Publishing.

West, D., & Marasco, L. (2009). *The breastfeeding mother's guide to making more milk.* New York, NY: McGraw Hill.

Equipment

Pumpin Pal
1–877–466–8283
www.pumpinpal.com/

Hands free pumping bras
http://www.handsfreepumpbra.com/
http://simplewishes.com/

Websites

Hand expressing and pumping videos
http://newborns.stanford.edu/Breastfeeding/

Low milk supply website
http://www.lowmilksupply.org/increasingmilk.shtml

Websites That Review Breast Pumps

http://www.breastpumpcomparisons.com/

www.amazon.com

www.epinions.com

References

Alekseev, N.P., Ilyin, V.I., Yaroslavski, V.K., Gaidukov, S.N., Tikhonova, T.K., Specivcev, Y.A., Omelyanjuk, E.V., & Tkachenko, N.N. (1998). Compression stimuli increase the efficacy of breast pump function. *European Journal of Obstetric Gynecologic and Reproductive Biology, 77,* 131–39.

Alekseev, N.P., Omel'ianuk, E.V., & Talalaeva, N.E. (2000). [Dynamics of milk ejection reflex during continuous rhythmic stimulation of areola-nipple complex of the mammary gland]. *Rossiiskii Fiziologicheskii Zhurnal Imeni I.M. Sechenova, 86,* 711–719.

Aljazaf, K.M.N.H. (2004). Ultrasound imaging in the analysis of the blood supply and blood flow in the human lactating breast. Dissertation. Perth, Australia: Medical Imaging Science, Curtin University of Technology.

Aljazaf, K., Hale, T.W., Ilett, K.F., Hartmann, P.E., Mitoulas, L.R., Kristensen, J.H., et al. (2003). Pseudoephedrine: effects on milk production in women and estimation of infant exposure via breastmilk. *British Journal of Clinical Pharmacology, 56,* 18–24.

Asquith, M.T., Sharp, R., & Stevenson, D.K. (1985). Decreased bacterial contamination of human milk expressed with an electric breast pump. *Journal of the California Perinatal Association, 4,* 45–47.

Atkinson, A. (2001). Decontamination of breast milk collection kits: a change in practice. *MIDIRS Midwifery Digest, 11,* 381–383.

Auerbach, K.G. (1990). Sequential and simultaneous breast pumping: a comparison. *International Journal of Nursing Studies, 27,* 257–265.

Barret, K.E., Barman, S.M., Boitano, S., et al. (2010). Immunity, infection and inflammation. In *Ganong's review of medical physiology* (23rd ed.; pp.63–78). McGraw-Hill, Lange, New York.

Berggren, K. (2006). *Working without weaning.* Amarillo, TX: Hale Publishing.

Biagioli, F. (2003). Returning to work while breastfeeding. *American Family Physician, 68,* 2199–2206.

Biancuzzo, (1999). Selecting pumps for breastfeeding mothers. *J Obstet Gynecol Neonatal Nurs, 28* (4), 417–426.

Binns, C.W., Win, N.N., Zhao, Y., & Scott, J.A. (2006). Trends in the expression of breastmilk 1993–2003. *Breastfeeding Review, 14,* 5–9.

Blenkharn, J.I. (1989). Infection risks from electrically operated breast pumps. *Journal of Hospital Infection, 13,* 27–31.

Boo, N.Y., Nordiah, A.J., Alfizah, H., & Nor-Rohaini, A.H. (2001). Contamination of breast milk obtained by manual expression and breast pump in mothers of very low birth weight infants. *Journal of Hospital Infection, 49,* 274–281.

Bowen-Jones, A., Thompson, C., & Drewett, R.F. (1982). Milk flow and sucking rates during breast-feeding. *Developmental Medicine and Child Neurology, 24,* 626–633.

Brown, S.L., Bright, R.A., Dwyer, D.E., & Foxman, B. (2005). Breast pump adverse events: reports to the Food and Drug Administration. *Journal of Human Lactation, 21,* 169–174.

Buckley, K.M. (2009). A double-edged sword: lactation consultants' perceptions of the impact of breast pumps on the practice of breastfeeding. *Journal of Perinatal Education, 18,* 13–22.

Caldeyro-Barcia R. (1969). Milk-ejection in women. In: Reynolds, M., & Folley. S. (eds.), *Lactogenesis, the initiation of milk secretion at parturition.* Philadelphia: University of Pennsylvania Press.

Carroll, L., Osman, M., Davies, D.P., & McNeish, A.S. (1979). Bacteriological criteria for feeding raw breast-milk to babies on neonatal units. *Lancet, 2*(8145), 732–733.

Chamberlain, L.B., McMahon, M., Philipp, B.L., & Merewood, A. (2006). Breast pump access in the inner city: a hospital-based initiative to provide breast pumps for low-income women. *Journal of Human Lactation, 22,* 94–98.

Chapman, D.J., Young, S., Ferris, A.M., & Pérez-Escamilla, R. (2001). Impact of breast pumping on lactogenesis stage II after cesarean delivery: a randomized clinical trial. *Pediatrics, 107,* e94.

Clark, A., & Dellaport, J. (2011). Development of a WIC single-user electric breast pump protocol. *Breastfeeding Medicine, 6,* 37–40.

Clavey, S. (1996). The use of acupuncture for the treatment of insufficient lactation (Que Ru). *American Journal of Acupuncture, 24,* 35–46.

Clemons, S.N., & Amir, L.H. (2010). Breastfeeding women's experience of expressing: a descriptive study. *Journal of Human Lactation, 26,* 258–265.

Clinical Lactation. (2011). Breastfeeding equipment to be allowed as medical tax deduction and reimbursed by flexible health spending accounts. *Clinical Lactation, 2,* 33.

Cobo, E., De Bernal, M.M., Gaitan, E., & Quintero, C.A. (1967). Neurohypophyseal hormone release in the human: II. Experimental study during lactation. *American Journal of Obstetrics and Gynecology, 97*, 519–29.

Cossey, V., Jeurissen, A., Thelissen, M.J., Vanhole, C., & Schuermans, A. (2011). Expressed breast milk on a neonatal unit: a hazard analysis and critical control points approach. *American Journal of Infection Control, 39*, 832–838.

Cotterman, K.J. (2004). Reverse pressure softening: a simple tool to prepare areola for easier latching during engorgement. *Journal of Human Lactation, 20*, 227–237.

Cox, D.B., Owens, R.A., & Hartmann, P.E. (1996). Blood and milk prolactin and the rate of milk synthesis in women. *Experimental Physiology, 81*, 1007–1020.

Cregan, M.D., De Mello, T.R., & Hartmann, P.E. (2000). Preterm delivery and breast expression: consequences for initiating lactation. *Advances Experimental Medicine Biology, 478*, 427–28.

Cregan, M.D., & Hartmann, P.E. (1999). Computerized breast measurement from conception to weaning: clinical implications. *Journal of Human Lactation, 15*, 89–96.

Daly, S.E.J., & Hartmann, P.E. (1995a). Infant demand and milk supply. Part 1: Infant demand and milk production in lactating women. *Journal of Human Lactation, 11*, 21–26.

Daly, S.E.J., & Hartmann, P.E. (1995b). Infant demand and milk supply. Part 2: The short-term control of milk synthesis in lactating women. *Journal of Human Lactation, 11*, 27–37.

Daly, S.E., Kent, J.C., Huynh, D.Q., Owens, R.A., Alexander, B.F., Ng, K.C., & Hartmann, P.E. (1992). The determination of short-term breast volume changes and the rate of synthesis of human milk using computerized breast measurement. *Experimental Physiology, 77*, 79–87.

Daly, S.E.J., Kent, J.C., Owens, R.A., & Hartmann, P.E. (1996). Frequency and degree of milk removal and the short-term control of human milk synthesis. *Experimental Physiology, 81*, 861–875.

Daly, S.E., Owens, R.A., & Hartmann, P.E. (1993). The short-term synthesis and infant regulated removal of milk in lactating women. *Experimental Physiology, 78*, 209–220.

de Sanctis, V., Vitali, U., Atti, G., Vullo, C., Sabato, A., & Bagni, B. (1981). Comparison of prolactin response to suckling and breast pump aspiration in lactating mothers. *La Ricerca in clinica e in laboratorio, 11*, 81–85.

Dewey, K.G., & Lonnerdal, B. (1986). Infant self-regulation of breast milk intake. *Acta Paediatrica Scandinavia, 75,* 893–898.

D'Amico, C.J., DiNardo, C.A., & Krystofiak, S. (2003). Preventing contamination of breast pump kit attachments in the NICU. *Journal of Perinatal and neonatal Nursing, 17,* 150–157.

DiPierro, F., Callegari, A., Carotenuto, D., & Tapia, M.M. (2008). Clinical efficacy, safety and tolerability of BIO-C (micronized silymarin) as a galactagogue. *Acta Biomedica, 79,* 205–210.

Donowitz, L.G., Marsik, F.J., Fisher, K.A., & Wenzel, R.P. (1981). Contaminated breast milk: a source of Klebsiella bacteremia in a newborn intensive care unit. *Reviews of Infectious Diseases, 3,* 716–720.

Drewett, R., Bowen-Jones, A., & Dogterom, J. (1982). Oxytocin levels during breastfeeding in established lactation. *Hormone Behavior, 16,* 245–248.

Egnell, E. (1956). Viewpoints on what happens mechanically in the female breast during various methods of milk collection. *Sven Lakartidn, 53,* 2553–2564.

Eidelman, A. I., & Szilagyi, G. (1979). Patterns of bacterial colonization of human milk. *Obstetrics and Gynecology, 53,* 550–552.

Engstrom, J.L., Meier, P.P., Jegier, B., Motykowski, J.E., & Zuleger, J.L. (2007). Comparison of milk output from the right and left breasts during simultaneous pumping in mothers of very low birthweight infants. *Breastfeeding Medicine, 2,* 83–91.

Faro, J., Katz, A., Berens, P., & Ross P.J. (2011). Premature termination of nursing secondary to *Serratia marcescens* breast pump contamination. *Obstetrics & Gynecology, 117,* 485–486.

Fewtrell, M.S., Loh, K.L., Blake, A., Ridout, D.A., & Hawdon, J. (2006). Randomised, double blind trial of oxytocin nasal spray in mothers expressing breast milk for preterm infants. *Archives of Disease in Children Fetal Neonatal Edition, 91,* F169-F174.

Fewtrell, M., Lucas, P., Collier, S., & Lucas, A. (2001). Randomized study comparing the efficacy of a novel manual breast pump with a mini-electric breast pump in mothers of term infants. *Journal of Human Lactation, 17,* 126–131.

Fewtrell, M.S., Lucas, P., Collier, S., Singhal, A., Ahluwalia, J.S., & Lucas, A. (2001). Randomized trial comparing the efficacy of a novel manual breast pump with a standard electric breast pump in mothers who delivered preterm infants. *Pediatrics, 107,* 1291–1297.

Fildes, V. (1986). *Breasts, bottles, and babies* (pp.141–143). Edinburgh: Edinburgh University.

Flaherman, V.J., Gay, B., Scott, C., Avins, A., Lee, K.A., & Newman, T.B. (2012). Randomised trial comparing hand expression with breast pumping for mothers of term newborns feeding poorly. *Archives of Disease in Children Fetal Neonatal Edition, 97,* F18-F23.

Foxman, B., D'Arcy, H., Gillespie, B., Bobo, J.K., & Schwartz, K. (2002). Lactation mastitis: occurrence and medical management among 946 breastfeeding women in the United States. *American Journal of Epidemiology, 155,* 103–114.

Freeman, M.E., Kanyicska, B., Lerant, A., & Nagy, G. (2000). Prolactin structure, function, and regulation of secretion. *Physiological Review, 80,* 1523–1631.

Furman, L., Minich, N., & Hack, M. (2002). Correlates of lactation in mothers of very low birth weight infants. *Pediatrics, 109,* e57.

Geddes, D.T., Kent, J.C., Mitoulas, L.R., & Hartmann, P.E. (2008). Tongue movement and intra-oral vacuum in breastfeeding infants. *Early Human Development, 84,* 471–477.

Geraghty, S., Davidson, B., Tabangin, M., & Morrow, A. (2011). Predictors of breastmilk expression by 1 month postpartum and influence on breastmilk feeding duration. *Breastfeeding Medicine, 6,* DOI: 10.1089/bfm.2011.0029 Ahead of print.

Geraghty, S.R., Khoury, J.C., & Kalkwarf, H.J. (2005). Human milk pumping rates of mothers of singletons and mothers of multiples. *Journal of Human Lactation, 21,* 413–420.

Gilks, J., Gould, D., & Price, E. (2007). Decontaminating breast pump collection kits for use on a neonatal unit: review of current practice and the literature. *Journal of Neonatal Nursing, 13,* 191–198.

Gransden, W.R., Webster, M., French, G.L., & Phillips, I. (1986). An outbreak of *Serratia marcescens* transmitted by contaminated breast pumps in a special care baby unit. *Journal of Hospital Infection, 7,* 149–154.

Greenwell, E.A., Wyshak, G., Ringer, S.A., Johnson, L.C., Rivkin, M.J., & Lieberman, E. (2012). Intrapartum temperature elevation, epidural use, and adverse outcome in term infants. *Pediatrics, 129,* e447-e454.

Groh-Wargo, S., Toth, A., Mahoney, K., Simonian, S., Wasser, T., & Rose, S. (1995). The utility of a bilateral breast pumping system for mothers of premature infants. *Neonatal Network, 14,* 31–36.

Hall, R.T., Mercer, A.M., Teasley, S.L., McPherson, D.M., Simon, S.D., Santos, S.R., Meyers, B.M., & Hipsh, N.E. (2002). A breastfeeding assessment score to evaluate the risk for cessation of breastfeeding by 7–10 days of age. *Journal of Pediatrics, 141,* 659–664.

Halverson, H.M. Mechanisms of early infant feeding. (1944). *Journal of General Psychiatry,* 64, 185–223.

Hartmann, P.E. (2002). New insights into breast physiology and breast expression and development of the Symphony breastpump. In: *Human lactation-the science of the art series.* CD, Baar, Switzerland: Medela AG, Medical Technology.

Hayes, D.K., Prince, C.B., Espinueva, V., Fuddy, L.J., Li, R., & Grummer-Strawn, L.M. (2008). Comparison of manual and electric breast pumps among WIC women returning to work or school in Hawaii. *Breastfeeding Medicine,* 3, 3–10.

Henly, S.J., Anderson, C.M., Avery, M.D., Hills-Bonczyk, S.G., Potter, S., & Duckett, L.J. (1995). Anemia and insufficient milk in first-time mothers. *Birth,* 22, 86–92.

Hill, P.D., Aldag, J.C., & Chatterton, R.T. (1996). The effect of sequential and simultaneous breast pumping on milk volume and prolactin levels: a pilot study. *Journal of Human Lactation,* 12, 193–199.

Hill, P.D., Aldag, J.C., & Chatterton, R.T. (2001). Initiation and frequency of pumping and milk production in mothers of non-nursing preterm infants. *Journal of Human Lactation,* 17, 9–11.

Hill, P.D., Aldag, J.C., & Chatterton, R.T. (1999). Effects of pumping style on milk production in mothers of non-nursing preterm infants. *Journal of Human Lactation,* 15, 209–216.

Hill, P.D., Aldag, J.C., Chatterton, R.T., & Zinaman, M. (2005).Comparison of milk output between mothers of preterm and term infants: the first 6 weeks after birth. *Journal of Human Lactation,* 21, 22–30.

Hill, P.D., Aldag, J.C., Demirtas, H., Naeem, V., Parker, N.P., Zinaman, M.J., & Chatterton, R.T. (2009). Association of serum prolactin and oxytocin with milk production in mothers of preterm and term infants. *Biological Research for Nursing,* 10, 340–349.

Hopkinson, J., & Heird, W. (2009). Maternal response to two electric breast pumps. *Breastfeeding Medicine,* 4, 17–23.

Howie, P.W., McNeilly, A.S., McArdle, T., Smart, L., & Houston, M. (1980). The relationship between suckling-induced prolactin response and lactogenesis. *Journal of Clinical Endocrinology and Metabolism,* 50, 670–73.

Hurst, N., & Meier, P.P. (2010). Chapter 13: Breastfeeding the preterm infant. In: Riordan, J., & Wambach, K. (eds.), *Breastfeeding and human lactation* (4th ed.). Boston: Jones and Bartlett Publishers.

Ingram, J.C., Woolridge, M.W., Greenwood, R.J., & McGrath, L. (1999). Maternal predictors of early breast milk output. *Acta Pediatrica, 88,* 493–499.

Jackson, E. (2011).Controversies in postpartum contraception: when is it safe to start oral contraceptives after childbirth? *Thrombosis Research, 127,* Suppl 3:S35-S39.

Jacobs, L.A., Dickinson, J.E., Hart, P.D., Doherty, D.A., & Faulkner, S.J. (2007). Normal nipple position in term infants measured on breastfeeding ultrasound. *Journal of Human Lactation, 23,* 52–59.

Jantarasaengaram, S., & Sreewapa, P. (2011). Effects of domperidone on augmentation of lactation following cesarean delivery at full term. *International Journal of Gynaecology and Obstetrics,* Dec 19. [Epub ahead of print].

Jenner, C., & Filshie, J. (2002). Galactorrhoea following acupuncture. *Acupuncture Medicine, 20,* 107–108.

Johnson, C.A. (1983). An evaluation of breast pumps currently available on the American market. *Clinical Pediatrics, 22,* 40–45.

Jones, E., Dimmock, P.W., & Spencer, S.A. (2001). A randomized controlled trial to compare methods of milk expression after preterm delivery. *Archives of Disease in Childhood Fetal and Neonatal Edition, 85,* F91-F95.

Jones, E., & Hilton, S. (2009). Correctly fitting breast shields are the key to lactation success for pump dependent mothers following preterm delivery. *Journal of Neonatal Nursing, 15,* 14–17.

Kent, J.C., Geddes, D.T., Hepworth, A.R., & Hartmann, P.E. (2011). Effect of warm breastshields on breast milk pumping. *Journal of Human Lactation, 27,* 331–338.

Kent, J.C., Mitoulas, L.R., Cregan, M.D., Geddes, D.T., Larsson, M., Doherty, D.A., & Hartmann, P.E. (2008). Importance of vacuum for breastmilk expression. *Breastfeeding Medicine, 3,* 11–19.

Kent, J.C., Ramsay, D.T., Doherty, D., Larsson, M., & Hartmann, P.E. (2003). Response of breasts to different stimulation patterns of an electric breast pump. *Journal of Human Lactation, 19,* 179–186.

Labiner-Wolfe, J., Fein, S.B., Shealy, K.R., & Wang, C. (2008). Prevalence of breast milk expression and associated factors. *Pediatrics, 122*, Suppl 2:S63-S68.

Lau, C. (2001). Effects of stress on lactation. *Pediatric Clinics of North America, 48*, 221–234.

Lawrence, R.A., & Lawrence, R.M. (2011). *Breastfeeding: a guide for the medical profession* (p. 261). Maryland Heights, MO: Elsevier Mosby.

Marasco, L. (2006). The impact of thyroid dysfunction on lactation. *Breastfeeding Abstracts, 25*, 9, 11–12.

Marasco, L., Marmet, C., & Shell, E. (2000). Polycystic ovary syndrome: a connection to insufficient milk supply? *Journal of Human Lactation, 16*,143–148.

McNeilly, A.S., Robinson, I.C., Houston, M.J., & Howie, P.W. (1983). Release of oxytocin and prolactin response to suckling. *British Medical Journal, 286*, 646–647.

Meier, P.P., Engstrom, J.L., Hurst, N.M., Ackerman, B., Allen, M., Motykowski, J.E., Zuleger, J.L., & Jegier, B.J. (2008). A comparison of the efficiency, efficacy, comfort, and convenience of two hospital-grade electric breast pumps for mothers of very low birthweight infants. *Breastfeeding Medicine, 3*, 141–150.

Meier, P.P., Engstrom, J.L., Janes, J.E., Jegier, B.J., & Loera, F. (2012). Breast pump suction patterns that mimic the human infant during breastfeeding: greater milk output in less time spent pumping for breast pump-dependent mothers with premature infants. *Journal of Perinatology, 32*, 103–110.

Meier, P., Engstrom, J., Mingolelli, S., Miracle, D., & Kiesling, S. (2004). The Rush Mothers' Milk Club: breastfeeding interventions for mothers with very-low-birth-weight infants. *Journal of Obstetric, Gynecologic and Neonatal Nursing, 33*, 164–174.

Meier, P., Motyhowski, J., & Zuleger, J. (2004). Choosing a correctly fitted breast shield for milk expression. *Medela Messenger, 21*, 8–9.

Meier,P., & Wilks, S. (1987). The bacteria in expressed mothers' milk. *American Journal of Maternal Child Nursing MCN, 12*, 420–423.

Mitoulas, L.R., Lai, C.T., Gurrin, L.C., Larsson, M., & Hartmann, P.E. (2002a). Effect of vacuum profile on breast milk expression using an electric breast pump. *Journal of Human Lactation, 18*, 353–360.

Mitoulas, L.R., Lai, C.T., Gurrin, L.C., Larsson, M., & Hartmann, P.E. (2002b). Efficacy of breast milk expression using an electric breast pump. *Journal of Human Lactation, 18,* 344–352.

Mizuno, K., & Ueda, A. (2006). Changes in sucking performance from nonnutritive sucking to nutritive sucking during breast- and bottle-feeding. *Pediatric Research, 59,* 728–731.

Moloney, A.C., Quoraishi , A.H., Parry, P., & Hall, V. (1987). A bacteriological examination of breast pumps. *Journal of Hospital Infection, 9,* 169–174.

Monaci, G., & Woolridge, M. (2011). Ultrasound video analysis for understanding of infant breastfeeding. Presented at the International Conference on Signal Processing, Belgium, September 2011.

Morrison. B., Ludington-Hoe, S., & Anderson, G.C. (2006). Interruptions to breastfeeding dyads on postpartum day 1 in a university hospital. *Journal of Obstetric Gynecologic and Neonatal Nursing, 35,* 709–716.

Morse, J., & Bottorff, J. (1988). The emotional experience of breast expression. *Journal of Nurse Midwifery, 33,* 165–170.

Morton, J. (2009). Is the use of breast pumps out of hand? Mothers who use 'hands-on' technique see increase in milk production. *AAP News, 30,* 14.

Morton, J., Hall, J.Y., Wong, R.J., Thairu, L., Benitz, W.E., & Rhine, W.D. (2009). Combining hand techniques with electric pumping increases milk production in mothers of preterm infants. *Journal of Perinatology, 29,* 757–764.

Morton, J., Wong, R.J., Hall, J.Y., Pang, W.W., Lai, C.T., Lui, J., Hartmann, P.E., & Rhine, W.D. (2012). Combining hand techniques with electric pumping increases the caloric content of milk in mothers of preterm infants. *Journal of Perinatology,* doi:10.1038/jp.2011.195.

Motil, K.J., Thotathuchery, M., Montandon, C.M., Hachey, D.L., Boutton, T.W., Klein, P.D., & Garza, C. (1994). Insulin, cortisol and thyroid hormones modulate maternal protein status and milk production and composition in humans. *Journal of Nutrition, 124,* 1248–1257.

Neifert, M., & Seacat, J. (1985). *Milk yield and prolactin rise with simultaneous breast pumping.* Presented at Ambulatory Pediatric Association Meeting, Washington, DC, May 7–10, 1985.

Neri, I., Allais, B., Vaccaro, V., Minniti, S., Airola, G., Schiapparelli, P., Benedetto, C., & Facchinetti, F. (2011). Acupuncture treatment as breastfeeding support: preliminary data. *Journal of Alternative and Complementary Medicine, 17,* 133–137.

Neville, M. (1983). Regulation of mammary development and lactation. In: Neville, M., & Neifert, M. (eds.). *Lactation: physiology, nutrition and breast-feeding*. New York: Plenum, 118.

Newburger, A.E. (2006). Cosmetic medical devices and their FDA regulation. *Archives of Dermatology, 142,* 225–228.

Noel, G., Suh, H., & Frantz, A. (1974). Prolactin release during nursing and breast stimulation in postpartum and nonpostpartum subjects. *Journal of Clinical Endocrinology and Metabolism, 38,* 413–423.

Noel-Weiss, J., Woodend, A.K., Peterson, W., Gibb, W., & Groll, D.L. (2011). An observational study of associations among maternal fluid during parturition, neonatal output, and breastfed newborn weight loss. *International Breastfeeding Journal, 6,* 9.

Ohyama, M., Watabe, H., & Hayasaka, T. (2010). Manual expression and electric breast pumping in the first 48 h after delivery. *Pediatrics International, 52,* 39–43.

Page-Wilson, G., Smith, P.C., & Welt, C.K. (2007). Short-term prolactin administration causes expressible galactorrhea but does not affect bone turnover: pilot data for a new lactation agent. *International Breastfeeding Journal, 2,* 10.

Parker, L.A., Sullivan, S., Krueger, C., Kelechi, T., & Mueller, M. (2012). Effect of early breast milk expression on milk volume and timing of lactogenesis stage II among mothers of very low birth weight infants: a pilot study. *Journal of Perinatology,* doi:10.1038/jp.2011.78.

Paul, V.K., Singh, M., Deorari, A.K., Pacheco, J., & Taneja, U. (1996). Manual and pump methods of expression of breast milk. *Indian Journal of Pediatrics, 63,* 87–92.

Philipp, B.L., Brown, E., & Merewood, A. (2000). Pumps for Peanuts: leveling the field in the neonatal intensive care unit. *Journal of Perinatology, 4,* 249–250.

Pittard, W.B., Geddes, K.M., Brown, S., Mintz, S., & Hulsey, T.C. (1991). Bacterial contamination of human milk: container type and method of expression. *American Journal of Perinatology, 8,* 25–27.

Potter, B. (2005). Women's experiences of managing mastitis. *Community Practitioner, 78,* 209–212.

Powe, C.E., Allen, M., Puopolo, K.M., Merewood, A., Worden, S., Johnson, L.C., Fleischman, A., & Welt, C.K. (2010). Recombinant human prolactin for the treatment of lactation insufficiency. *Clinical Endocrinology (Oxf), 73,* 645–653.

Powe, C.E., Puopolo, K.M., Newburg, D.S., Lönnerdal, B., Chen, C., Allen, M., Merewood, A., Worden, S., & Welt, C.K. (2011). Effects of recombinant human prolactin on breast milk composition. *Pediatrics, 127*, e359–366.

Prime, D.K., Geddes, D.T., Hepworth, A.R., Trengove, N.J., & Hartmann, P.E. (2011). Comparison of the patterns of milk ejection during repeated breast expression sessions in women. *Breastfeeding Medicine, 6*, 183–190.

Prime, D.K., Geddes, D.T., Spatz, D.L., Robert, M., Trengove, N.J., & Hartmann, P.E. (2009). Using milk flow rate to investigate milk ejection in the left and right breasts during simultaneous breast expression in women. *International Breastfeeding Journal, 4,*10.

Prime, D.K., Kent, J.C., Hepworth, A.R., Trengove, N.J., & Hartmann, P.E. (2011). Dynamics of milk removal during simultaneous breast expression in women. *Breastfeeding Medicine,* Advance online publication DOI: 10.1089/bfm.2011.001

Ramsay, D.T., Mitoulas, L.R., Kent, J.C., Cregan, M.D., Doherty, D.A., Larsson, M., & Hartmann, P.E. (2006). Milk flow rates can be used to identify and investigate milk ejection in women expressing breast milk using an electric breast pump. *Breastfeeding Medicine 1*, 14–23.

Ramsay, D.T., Mitoulas, L.R., Kent, J.C., Larsson, M., & Hartmann, P.E. (2005). The use of ultrasound to characterize milk ejection on women using an electric breast pump. *Journal of Human Lactation, 21*, 421–428.

Roche-Paull, R. (2010). *Breastfeeding in combat boots: a survival guide to successful breastfeeding while serving in the military.* Amarillo, TX: Hale Publishing.

Schwartz, K., d'Arcy, H.J.S., Gillespie, B., Bobo, J., Longeway, M.L., & Foxman, B. (2002). Factors associated with weaning in the first 3 months postpartum. *Journal of Family Practice, 51*, 439–444.

Scientific American. (1863). *Scientific American, 8*(10), 156. New York.

Scientific American. (1863). *Scientific American, 8*(4), 49. New York.

Sharma, S., Ramji, S., Kumari, S., & Bapna, J.S. (1996). Randomised controlled trial of Asparagus racemosus (Shtavari) as a lactogogue in lactational inadequacy. *Indian Journal of Pediatrics, 33*, 675–677.

Sisk, P., Quandt, S., Parson, N., & Tucker, J. (2010). Breast milk expression and maintenance in mothers of very low birth weight infants: supports and barriers. *Journal of Human Lactation, 26*, 368–375.

Slusher, T., Slusher, I.L., Biomdo, M., Bode-Thomas, F., Curtis, B.A., & Meier, P. (2007). Electric breast pump use increases maternal milk volume in African nurseries. *Journal of Tropical Pediatrics, 53,* 125–30.

Slusher, T.M., Slusher, I.L., Keating, E.M., Curtis, B.A., Smith, E.A., Orodriyo, E., Awori, S., & Nakakeeto, M.K. (2011). Comparison of maternal milk (breastmilk) expression methods in an African nursery. *Breastfeeding Medicine, Jul 8.* [Epub ahead of print].

Smith, W., Erenberg, A., & Nowak, A. (1988). Imaging evaluation of the human nipple during breastfeeding. *American Journal of Disease in Children, 142,* 76–78.

Sozmen, M. (1992). Effects of early suckling of cesarean-born babies on lactation. *Biology of the Neonate, 62,* 67–68.

Stark, Y. (1994). Human nipples: function and anatomical variations in relationship to breastfeeding [master's thesis]. Pasadena, CA: Pacific Oaks College.

Stern, J.M., & Reichlin, S. (1990). Prolactin circadian rhythm persists throughout lactation in women. *Neuroendocrinology, 51,* 31–37.

Thom, A.R., Cole, A.P., & Watrasiewicz, K. (1970). *Pseudomonas aeruginosa* infection in a neonatal nursery possibly transmitted by a breast-milk pump. *Lancet, 1,* 560–561.

Thompson, N., Pickler, R.H., Munro, C., & Shotwell, J. (1997). Contamination in expressed breast milk following breast cleansing. *Journal of Human Lactation, 13,* 127–130.

Turkyilmaz, C., Onal, E., Hirfanoglu, I.M., Turan, O., Koc, E., Ergenekon, E., & Atalay, Y. (2011). The effect of galactagogue herbal tea on breast milk production and short-term catch-up of birth weight in the first week of life. *Journal of Alternative and Complementary Medicine, 17,* 139–142.

Tyson, J.E., Edwards, W.H., Rosenfeld, A.M., & Beer, A.E. (1982). Collection methods and contamination of bank milk. *Archives of Disease in Childhood, 57,* 396–398.

Walker, M. (1992). Breast pump survey. Unpublished manuscript.

Walker, M. (2009). *Breastfeeding the late preterm infant: improving care and outcomes.* Amarillo, TX: Hale Publishing.

Walker, M. (2011). *Breastfeeding and employment: making it work.* Amarillo, TX: Hale Publishing.

Wan, E.W., Davey, K., Page-Sharp, M., Hartmann, P.E., Simmer, K., & Ilett, K.F. (2008). Dose-effect study of domperidone as a galactagogue in preterm

Index

mothers with insufficient milk supply, and its transfer into milk. *British Journal of Clinical Pharmacology, 66,* 283–289.

Weber, F., Woolridge, M.W., & Baum, J.D. (1986). An ultrasonographic study of the organization of sucking and swallowing by newborn infants. *Developmental Medicine and Child Neurology, 28,* 19–24.

Wei, L., Wang, H., Han, Y., & Li, C. (2008). Clinical observation on the effects of electroacupuncture at Shaoze (SI 1) in 46 cases of postpartum insufficient lactation. *Journal of Traditional Chinese Medicine, 28,* 168–172.

Weichert, C. (1980). Prolactin cycling and the management of breastfeeding failure. *Advances in Pediatrics, 27,* 391–407.

West, D., & Marasco, L. (2009). *The breastfeeding mother's guide to making more milk.* New York: McGraw Hill.

Whittlestone, W. (1978). The physiologic breastmilker. *New Zealand Family Physician, 5,* 1–3.

Wight, N., Turfler, K., Grassley, J., & Spencer, B. (2011). Evaluation of milk production with a multi-user, electric double pump with a soft flange in mothers of very low birth weight (VLBW) (<1500gm, <31 wk gest) NICU infants: a pilot study. *Breastfeeding Medicine, 6,* Suppl 1, S21-S22.

Wiklund. I., Norman, M., Uvnäs-Moberg, K., Ransjö-Arvidson, A.B., & Andolf, E. (2009). Epidural analgesia: breast-feeding success and related factors. *Midwifery, 25,* e31–38.

Wilde, C.J., Prentice, A., & Peaker, M. (1995). Breast-feeding: matching supply with demand in human lactation. *Proceedings of the Nutrition Society, 54,* 401–406.

Wilks, S., & Meier, P. (1988). Helping mothers express milk suitable for preterm and high-risk infant feeding. *American Journal of Maternal Child Nursing MCN, 13,* 121–123.

Wilson-Clay, B., & Hoover, K. (2002). *The breastfeeding atlas* (2nd ed.). Austin, TX: LactNews Press.

Wilson-Clay, B., & Hoover, K. (2005). *The breastfeeding atlas* (3rd ed.). Austin, TX: LactNews Press.

Win, N.N., Binns, C.W., Zhao, Y., Scott, J.A., & Oddy, W.H. (2006). Breastfeeding duration in mothers who express breast milk: a cohort study. *International Breastfeeding Journal, 1,* 28.

Woolridge, M.W. (1995). Breastfeeding: physiology into practice. In: Davies, D.P. (ed.), *Nutrition in child health. Proceedings of conference jointly organized by the Royal College of Physicians of London and the British Paediatric Association* (pp.13–31). RCPL Press.

Woolridge, M. (2011). The mechanisms of breastfeeding revised-new insights into how babies feed provided by a fresh ultrasound studies of breastfeeding. *Evidence-based Child Health 6,* (Suppl. 1), 46.

Yigit, F., Cigdem, Z., Temizsoy, E., Cingi, M.E., Korel, O., Yildirim, E., & Ovali, F. (2012). Does warming the breasts affect the amount of breastmilk production? *Breastfeeding Medicine,* Mar 16. [Epub ahead of print].

Yokoyama, Y., Ueda, T., Irahara, M., & Aono, T. (1994). Releases of oxytocin and prolactin during breast massage and suckling in puerperal women. *European Journal of Obstetrics and Gynecology and Reproductive Biology, 53,* 17–20.

Zhao, Y., & Guo, H. (2006). The therapeutic effects of acupuncture in 30 cases of postpartum hypogalactia. *Journal of Traditional Chinese Medicine, 26,* 29–30.

Zhou, H.Y., Li, L., Li, D., Li, X., Meng, H.J., Gao, X.M., et al. (2009). Clinical observation on the treatment of post-cesarean hypogalactia by auricular points sticking-pressing. *Chinese Journal of Integrative Medicine, 15,* 117–120.

Ziemer, M.M., & Pigeon, J.G. (1993). Skin changes and pain in the nipple during the 1st week of lactation. *Journal of Obstetric Gynecologic Neonatal Nursing, 22,* 247–256.

Zinaman, M. (1988). Breast pumps: ensuring mothers' success. *Contemporary Obstetrics and Gynecology, 32,* 55–62.

Zinaman, M.J., Hughes, V., Queenan, J.T., Labbok, M.H., & Albertson, B. (1992). Acute prolactin and oxytocin responses and milk yield to infant suckling and artificial methods of expression in lactating women. *Pediatrics, 89,* 437–440.

Zoppou, C., Barry, S.I., & Mercer, G.N. (1997a). Dynamics of human milk extraction: a comparative study of breast feeding and breast pumping. *Bulletin of Mathematical Biology, 59,* 953–73.

Zoppou, C., Barry, S.I., & Mercer, G.N. (1997b). Comparing breastfeeding and breast pumps using a computer model. *Journal of Human Lactation, 13,* 195–202.

Zuppa, A.A., Sindico, P., Orchi, C., Carducci, C., Cardiello, V., & Romagnoli, C. (2010). Safety and efficacy of galactogogues: substances that induce, maintain and increase breast milk production. *Journal of Pharmacy and Pharmaceutical Science, 13,* 162–174.

About the Author

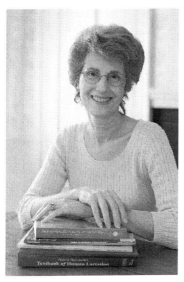

Marsha Walker, RN, IBCLC is the Executive Director of the National Alliance for Breastfeeding Advocacy, Research, Education and Legal Branch (NABA REAL). She is a long time breastfeeding advocate, starting as a volunteer breastfeeding counselor with the Nursing Mothers Counsel in California. Marsha went on to become a childbirth educator through Lamaze International, a registered nurse, and an International Board Certified Lactation Consultant. She served on the Representative Panel of Experts in 1985, which constructed the first lactation consultant exam and was one of a number of clinicians on whose practice the exam grid is based. Marsha enjoyed a large clinical lactation practice at Harvard Pilgrim Health Plan, a major HMO in Massachusetts, where she was the Director of the Breastfeeding Support Program for 12 years. She has served on the Board of Directors of the International Lactation Consultant Association (ILCA) for 7 years, including as its president in 1999.

Marsha is on the Board of Directors of the Massachusetts Breastfeeding Coalition, Baby Friendly USA, the US Lactation Consultant Association, and Best for Babes. She is ILCA's representative to the US Department of Agriculture's Breastfeeding Promotion Consortium and NABA's representative to the US Breastfeeding Committee. She has worked for 8 years to get breastfeeding legislation passed in her state of Massachusetts, which became a reality in January 2009. She is the co-chair of the Ban the Bags campaign, a national effort to eliminate the hospital distribution of formula company discharge bags.

NABA REAL is the IBFAN organization in the United States and is responsible for monitoring the International Code of Marketing of Breastmilk Substitutes in the US. Marsha has written both country reports on Code monitoring activities in the US, "Selling Out Mothers and Babies" and "Still Selling Out Mothers and Babies." Marsha is an international speaker on breastfeeding and an author of numerous publications, including her book "Breastfeeding Management for the Clinician: Using the Evidence."

Marsha is married and the mother of two breastfed children, Shannon and Justin, her original breastfeeding clinical instructors. She is the grandmother of 4 breastfed girls - Haley, Sophie, Isabelle, and Ella.

Made in the USA
Middletown, DE
19 September 2019